AMAZING SMILES

THROUGH COSMETIC DENTISTRY

BY ALBERT J. KURPIS, D.D.S.

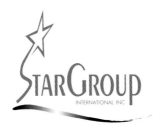

DEDICATION

To my best friend and love of my life, my wife, Judy,
who is always there to provide me with never ending support.

And to my three children, Jonathan, Lauren and Brian,
who have grown up to be very special young adults.

FIRST EDITION

Production by StarGroup International, Inc.
West Palm Beach, Florida
(561) 547-0667
www.stargroupinternational.com

Edited by Shawn McAllister

Cover and book designed by Mel Abfier

Printed in Korea

Library of Congress Cataloging-in-Publication Data pending

Amazing Smiles Through Cosmetic Dentstry, Albert J. Kurpis, D.D.S.

ISBN 1-884886-80-9

Legal Statement

The information contained in this book is for informational purposes only. It is not a substitute for professional advice provided by a dentist or physician. The intention of this book is to be a reference source only, which allows you to communicate more effectively with your dentist when making decisions about your dental care. No information within this book is intended to constitute a medical or dental diagnosis or treatment or endorsement of any particular test or procedure or service, etc. Reliance on any information in this book is at the reader's own risk. No information within this book is intended in any way to interfere with the diagnosis or treatment, past or present, of any patient by any physician or dentist. Although efforts are made to include information that is accurate, no representations or warranties regarding errors, omissions, completeness, or accuracy of information is provided. No action should be taken by you or any other individual based on any information contained within this book without the advice of a licensed dentist. If you suspect you have a dental or medical problem, you should immediately seek the advice of a dentist or physician. The author expressly disclaims any responsibility for any adverse effects whether physical or psychological, occurring as a result of any use of this book or use of any information within this book. If you do not understand and agree with this legal statement, please do not read this book.

TABLE OF CONTENTS

ACKNOWLEDGEMENTS

There are so many people who have contributed
to making this book possible. I particularly want to thank
Brenda Star, President of Star Group International for encouraging me
to go forward with this project. I also want to thank her great
editor, Shawn McAllister and talented designer, Mel Abfier.
As with so many projects, there are so many people in the background
on whose support I could always count. They include my associates,
Dr. John Ianzano and Dr. John Varoscak. In addition, my great staff was
always there to help with the details. Thanks Kristine, Liz, Karen, Francy,
Alma, Barbara, Debbie, Nancy, Sarah and Katherine. A special thanks to
my wife, Judy and my daughter, Lauren, for all those countless hours
they spent editing my final draft. My daughter, Lauren, who is finishing
her training at Columbia University, College of Dental Medicine, was an
invaluable source of help and insight with the more technical aspects of
this book. Finally, I would like to acknowledge the outstanding work by
Danny, Glen, CK, Charlie and all the other technicians at Americus Lab
who made most of these cases possible.
And let us not forget the master ceramist, the late Yasuo Saita,
the genius behind so many great smiles.

INTRODUCTION

What is Cosmetic Dentistry?

Welcome to the world of Amazing Smiles! For the very first time in human history, man has the ability to dramatically improve his appearance through the marvels of cosmetic dentistry. Cosmetic dentistry, simply stated, is the art and science of a person's teeth and smile, thereby changing someone's entire appearance.

The field of dentistry developed in response to a human need. That need was to correct all ailments associated with teeth and gums. This included restoring or replacing broken or missing teeth.

Dentistry's primary goal is still to restore a patient's overall oral health. While physical health is always the main objective of dentistry, another need emerged concerning our teeth; we developed a desire to look more attractive.

We all want and need to feel good about ourselves. Nowhere is that more important than at the most apparent focal point of our faces… our smile. Our smile reveals so much about us. It communicates our intentions. It lets others know if we approve, if we like, or if we are attracted to what we observe. On the other hand, when we believe that our smile is a detriment, it can dramatically alter how effectively we are able to communicate. When we lose our ability to communicate, our life changes. Some people believe in their hearts that they never had the ability to communicate effectively because they never had an attractive smile. For these people, an unattractive smile can have incredible negative consequences that affect self-esteem. An unattractive smile affects people both in social situations and in their job performance.

We are often not aware of how people around us react to our smile. Does anyone doubt that a smile is not that important? Imagine making an expensive purchase of an elegant product or high end service from someone with a horrific smile. How do you think this would affect you? Would it enhance or detract from this special experience? What would happen in a restaurant if you notice that your waiter has infected gums and horrible teeth? You just may lose your appetite. What about meeting that special someone in your life? Your eyes meet. Then the subliminal smile says something… what would yours say if you did not like your own smile?

Unfortunately, people with unattractive teeth and gums tend to hide their smile. Some people withdraw from situations that could possibly expose their unsightly smile. Some lack the confidence to take the lead and/or project their views in front of others because they imagine that they may be judged by their smile. Often they are not as effective as they could be in business situations, social encounters or romantic relations. Some of these people become more introverted and, at times, depressed. They avoid social interactions for fear of rejection or embarrassment. Patients in their 50s and early 60s who have worn or dark teeth start to look and feel prematurely older than they really are. This may be the catalyst of a winding downward spiral into old age.

As sad as all this may seem, it does not have to be this way. There is hope and there are real solutions. With advances in modern cosmetic dentistry, a mouth can be restored so that any person suffering from low self-esteem can become more confident. A bright, new smile can literally change one's life.

This book will become an invaluable tool to anyone looking to benefit from a better looking smile. But first, there are some things you must know.

Welcome to the life changing field of cosmetic dentistry. Cosmetic dentistry is that area of dentistry that not only restores teeth to a state of health, but also emphasizes and improves the appearance of a smile. Cosmetic dentistry should be regarded both as an art and a science with the objective of making one's smile more beautiful. With the aid of the latest materials and techniques, cosmetic dentistry can change and create a better looking smile more comfortably than ever before.

The following chapters provide the rules that govern how smiles look, show the procedures that can be used to attain an attractive smile, demonstrate real life examples of these procedures and answer the most frequently asked questions regarding cosmetic dentistry. My intention is to inspire you or someone important in your life to get on the road to a healthy and amazing smile.

Cosmetic Dentistry from the Beginning

Throughout human history, the importance of caring for teeth and enhancing the individual smile has been important. As early as 3000-2500 B.C., the procedures for saving teeth were evidenced by skulls found containing teeth connected together with gold wires. The smile was so important that wealthy Egyptians even depicted their smiles on golden mummy masks found in ancient tombs (photo 1). Primitive fixed dental bridges made from gold bands and human teeth have been found on Etruscan skulls in what is now Tuscany, Italy, as early as 500 B.C.

Polished semi-precious stones and sea shells have been found implanted into the jaw bones of early Pre-Columbian Indians throughout the Americas. Gold appliances found on skulls may have been used to strengthen loose teeth or improve the cosmetic appearance of these ancient people. Cosmetic enhancement of Mayan teeth was performed by placing semi-precious stones in the middle of the upper and lower teeth (photo 2).

The Persian Middle Ages were also a time of advances in cosmetic dentistry. Teeth made of ivory have been found implanted in skulls of the wealthier classes. The first known set of removable false teeth was fabricated during the six-

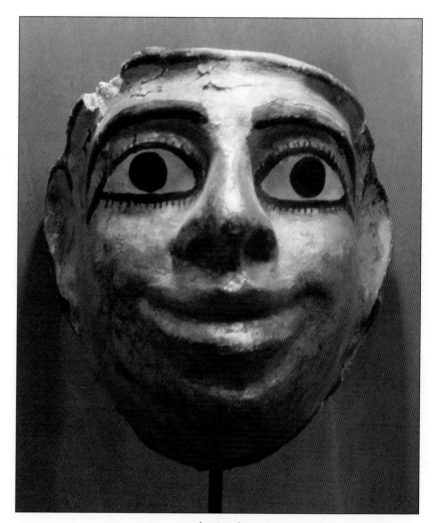

photo 1

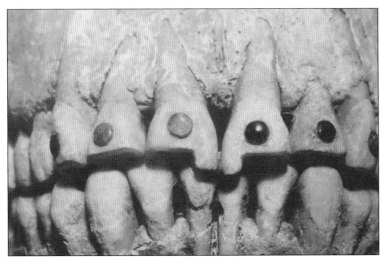

photo 2

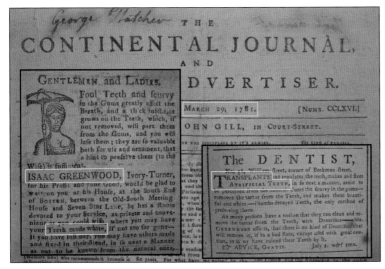

photo 3

teenth century. By the 18th century, false teeth made of ivory and human teeth were in widespread use among the aristocracy. These advances were advertised in local newspapers.

Cosmetic dental procedures aimed at improving smiles continued to be performed during the 18th and 19th centuries. In 1789, the very first American born dentist, Dr. Isaac Greenwood, placed advertisements in the Boston newspaper, The Continental Journal, advertising his cosmetic dental procedures. His son, Dr. John Greenwood, who later became famous for being George Washington's dentist, advertised his tooth transplant procedure as well (photo 3). By the early 20th century, dental materials and techniques improved, bringing costs down and making cosmetic dentistry available to the growing middle class. More people could now take advantage of cosmetic dental procedures. As demand for these procedures increased, many dentists started to devote their entire practice to cosmetic dentistry. These professionals became known as Cosmetic Dentists.

With the establishment of the American Academy of Cosmetic Dentistry and the growing popularity of cosmetic procedures, cosmetic dentistry became a focal point in American culture. As 20th century culture evolved, new emphasis was placed on beauty and appearance. Nowhere else was it noted more than in the American smile. In magazines, in movies, and on television shows, our media icons were all displaying that attractive "Hollywood Smile." By the 21st century, cosmetic makeover reality shows brought cosmetic dentistry procedures into our homes. The era of the AMAZING SMILE emerged.

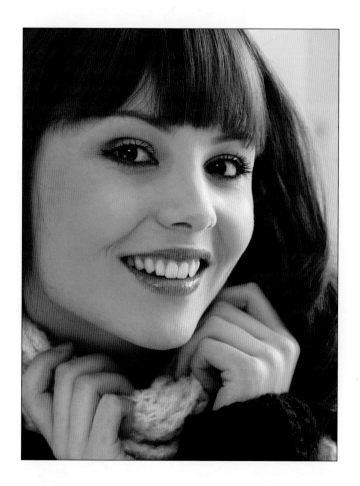

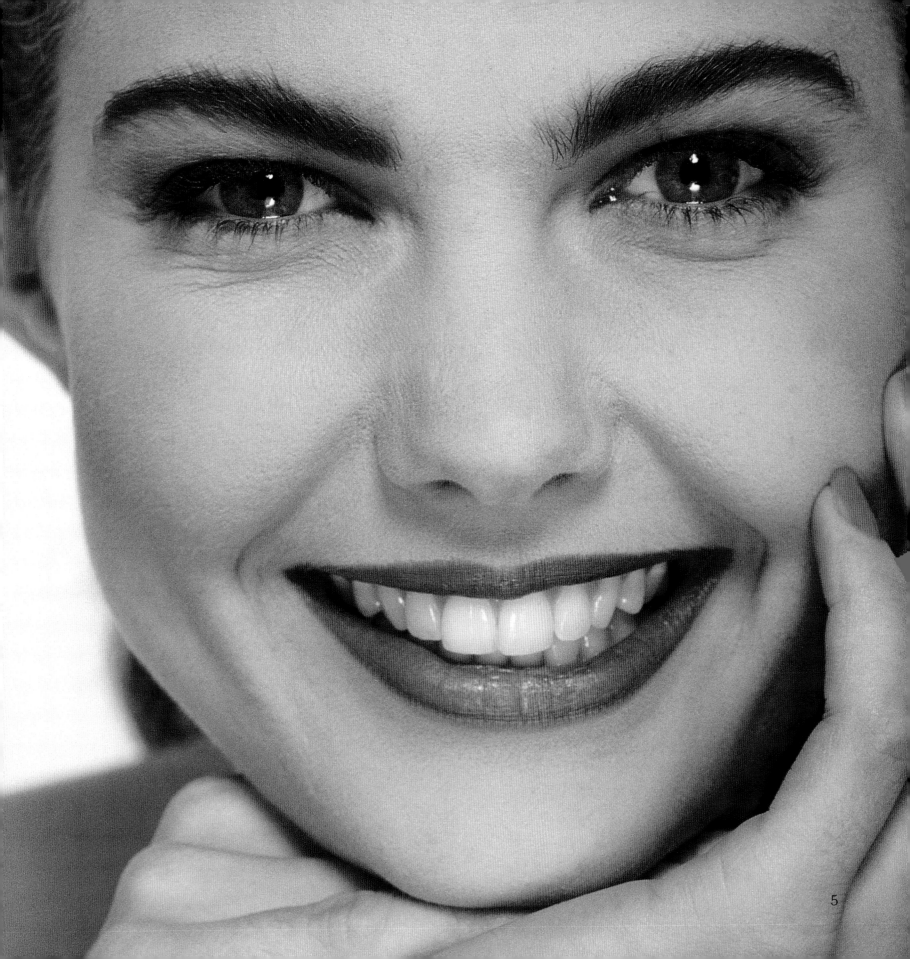

Factors that Determine How Your Smile Looks

A great looking smile creates an illusion of energy. While it seems that people with attractive and alluring smiles all have big, white, straight teeth, closer examination reveals that people with great looking smiles do not necessarily have the same perfect teeth. Beautiful teeth come in a wide variety of shapes, sizes, arrangements and colors that suit each person's face individually.

Like a fine oil painting, each smile is a canvas containing the application of many elements, and the unique relationship of these elements to each other. Just as an artist combines elements to create a painting that is pleasing to the eye, a cosmetic dentist chooses elements for teeth that will produce the perfect smile. Just as no two paintings are alike, no two smiles are the same.

Many choices and variations must be considered in creating a beautiful smile. The patient's own perception of beauty must be taken into consideration. By combining the art and science of smile design with the patient's desires, an aesthetically pleasing smile can be created. Although science dictates the methodology used, the procedure is an artistic creation. The process is a collaboration between doctor and patient. In order for the process of smile creation to be suc-

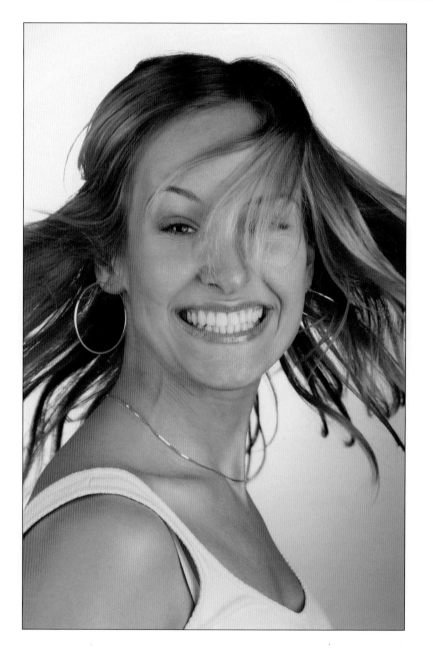

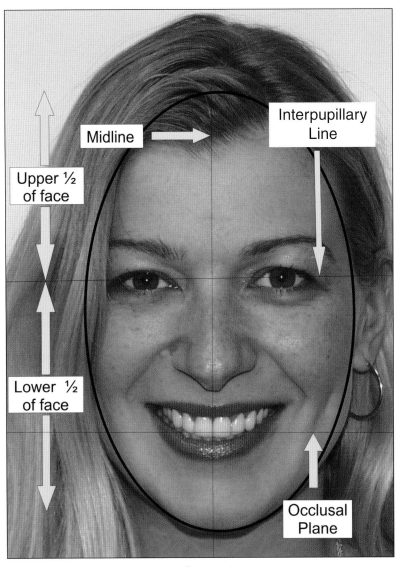

Midline

Interpupillary Line

Upper ½ of face

Lower ½ of face

Occlusal Plane

figure 1

cessful, it is absolutely essential that excellent communication exists between the cosmetic dentist and the patient.

Average patients usually have little or no knowledge about cosmetic dentistry. They may know what they like or don't like, but they may not know why. Here are the basics of cosmetic dentistry and the principles that guide visual appearance.

Everyone possesses certain basic facial characteristics. There are specific fundamentals that apply to the human head. For example, the human head is approximately an oval. The eyes are located on a horizontal plane that bisects the head into two halves; the upper half and the lower half (figure 1). This bisecting line, called the interpupillary line, connects the pupils of the eyes. The interpupillary line connecting the centers of the eyes establishes a reference point for the horizontal center of the face. Other facial features, including teeth, are balanced with it. When viewed from the front of a face, the horizontal plane of the teeth are parallel to this line. This parallel alignment is known as the frontal view occlusal plane or plane of occlusion of the teeth.

The most important vertical line on the face is the midline, which divides the face vertically into two halves. The center of the two front, upper teeth (the upper incisors) most commonly lines up with the midline of the face.

The nose plays an important part in the creative decision making process. When the nose is crooked or off to one side, the decision needs to be made whether the center of the teeth look better centered with the midline of the face or centered with the bottom of the base of the nose (figure 2). Both situations can work on different people. It's up to patients to decide what better suits them.

Many times, the teeth are the correct shape, size and color, but the plane of occlusion is off on one side. The plane is either too high or too low, making the teeth appear as though they are slanting or running up hill or down hill when observed in a mirror.

To achieve a well balanced smile, any discrepancy between the occlusal plane and the interpupillary line must be corrected as much as possible (figure 3).

If one eye is significantly higher than the other, the teeth must be balanced with the mouth. Here is where the "art" of cosmetic dentistry comes into play.

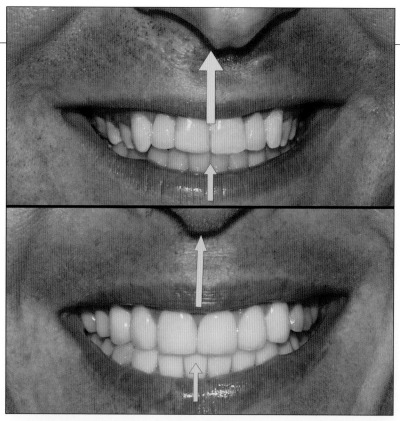

figure 2

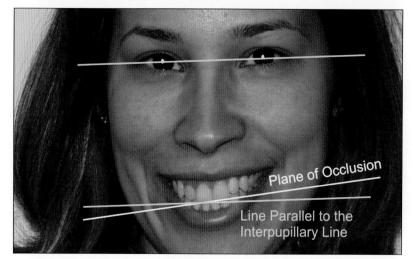

figure 3

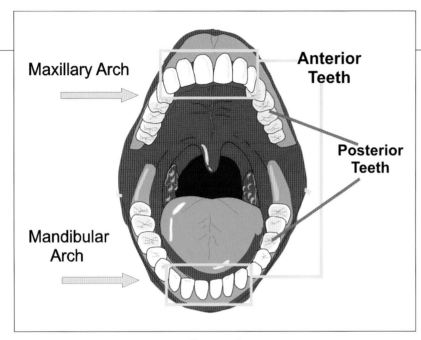

figure 4

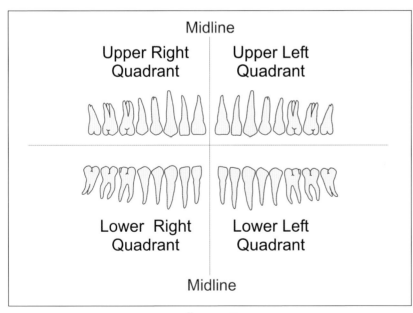

figure 5

If you as a patient want to achieve a particular aesthetic look that you believe is correct for your face, you must be able to communicate clearly with your cosmetic dentist about your smile and the teeth within your mouth. In order to do that, you must understand how teeth are arranged and what terminology is used to describe them.

The mouth consists of the upper (maxillary) jaw and the lower (mandibular) jaw. The teeth of each jaw are arranged in an arch and are referred to as the upper (maxillary) arch and the lower (mandibular) arch. The front teeth in both arches from canine to canine (the 3rd tooth from the midline) are called the anterior teeth. All the teeth behind the canines are called the posterior teeth (figure 4).

When viewing an entire mouth we see that the teeth are also divided into four groups or quadrants. Viewed from the front, they are identified as the upper right quadrant, the upper left quadrant, the lower right quadrant and the lower left quadrant (figure 5). Using descriptive quadrant terminology helps locate teeth in general areas of the mouth. This quadrant terminology is used when giving feedback to your cosmetic dentist.

There are 32 individual teeth in the adult dentition. For reference purposes, they are each assigned a number from 1 to 32 (figure 6). The number 1 tooth starts with the last tooth in the upper right quadrant and continues numerically forward around the arch to the back of the upper left quadrant to the number 16. The numbering system continues down to the back of the lower left quadrant to number 17 and continues forward to the last tooth in the lower right quadrant, number 32. When teeth are entered into a computer or information about them is sent to an insurance company, they are referred to by their numbers. If teeth are missing from the arch, their spaces on the arch are still referred to by their numbers. For example, if tooth number 4 is missing but was going to be replaced by a dental implant, you would say that the implant was being placed in area number 4.

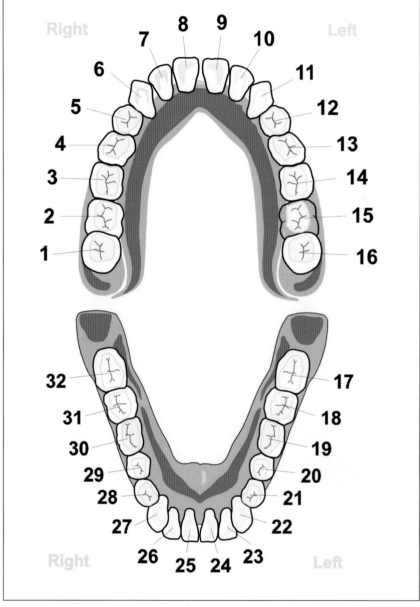

figure 6

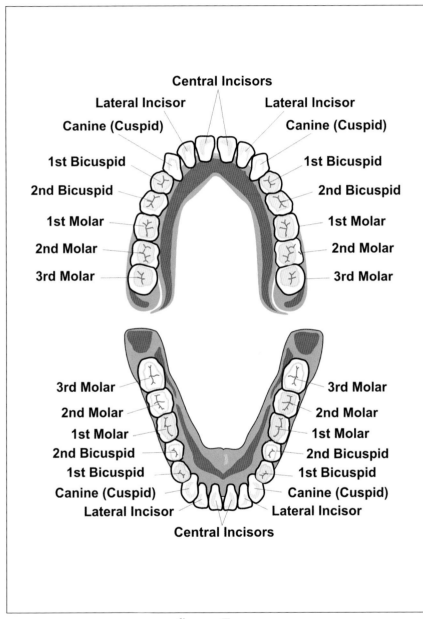

Central Incisors
Lateral Incisor   Lateral Incisor
Canine (Cuspid)   Canine (Cuspid)
1st Bicuspid   1st Bicuspid
2nd Bicuspid   2nd Bicuspid
1st Molar   1st Molar
2nd Molar   2nd Molar
3rd Molar   3rd Molar

3rd Molar   3rd Molar
2nd Molar   2nd Molar
1st Molar   1st Molar
2nd Bicuspid   2nd Bicuspid
1st Bicuspid   1st Bicuspid
Canine (Cuspid)   Canine (Cuspid)
Lateral Incisor   Lateral Incisor
Central Incisors

figure 7

Although all teeth are assigned numbers, they are more commonly referred to by their names (figure 7). These names are used by patients and dentists to discuss how they look in the mouth. For more accurate descriptions of a tooth, a location name is used before the name of the tooth is given. For example, when referring to the arch in which teeth are found, the terms maxilla and mandible are used to describe the upper and lower jaws, respectively. The first location name is followed by a descriptive second name. The descriptive second name relates to its function in the mouth. The names of the front four teeth are called incisors, so these incisors are referred to as the maxillary and mandibular incisors. The function of the incisors is to tear, penetrate, and incise food in the mouth. Incisors are arranged in groups of four. They are the central incisors and the lateral incisors. On each side of the incisors are the canines (also called cuspids).

After the anterior teeth (consisting of incisors and canines) are the posterior teeth, known as the first bicuspids, second bicuspids, first molars, second molars and third molars (wisdom teeth). As teeth are discussed and described, you can see how complex yet accurate this teminology may appear. For example, tooth number 14 is described as the left maxillary first molar. Tooth number 25 is the right mandibular central incisor.

This may sound confusing in the beginning, but once the numbers and names become familiar the whole oral naming system will make perfect sense.

A tooth is much more than a number, a location or a name; it is a living entity within the jawbone. It has very specific macro and micro anatomy. The anatomy of a tooth is very complex, which is the reason why dentists spend a minimum of four to five years studying dentistry before they have the opportunity to create smiles for patients. For the sake of simplicity, here is a very brief explanation of tooth anatomy (figure 8).

The part of the tooth that can be seen in the mouth is called the crown. The part that cannot be seen, below the crown and in the jaw bone, is the root. The crown of a tooth consists of a hard outer shell, called the enamel. This is a crystallized structure giving a tooth its hardness, characteristic look and color. Under the enamel is a softer hard layer called the dentin. The color of the dentin may also influence the color of the overlying enamel covering. Within the dentin lies a space occupied by arteries, veins and nerve tissue called the dental pulp, commonly referred to as the nerve. This nerve extends all the way to the bottom of the root of the tooth. Each tooth is attached to the surrounding bone by a soft tissue called the periodontal ligament. Covering the bone and surrounding the base of each tooth is a soft pink tissue called the gingiva (commonly known as the gums).

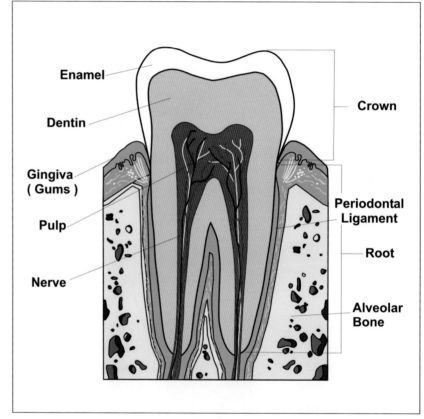

figure 8

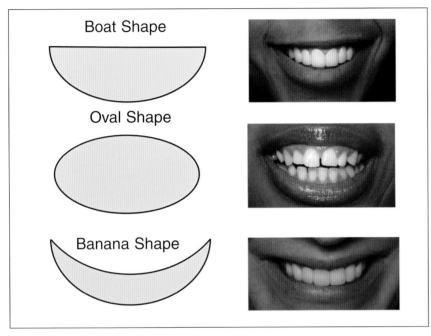

figure 9

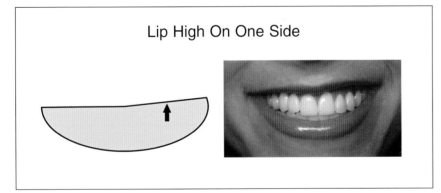

figure 10

Now that we have a basic understanding of what a tooth is, where it is, and what its parts are called, let's look at the overall smile (figure 9).

The lips determine the general shape of the mouth when a smile is formed. Some smiles have the shape of a boat, and others look like an oval or a banana. No matter how the teeth are arranged or changed, the lips are the overall curtain that frames the teeth and influences the look of a smile. Many times, patients produce pictures, saying, "I want to look like him/her." The reality is that they can't. The problem is that these patients do not understand that they have completely different shaped lips and mouths. Unless lips, shapes of mouths or arch forms are noted and discussed at the beginning of the consultation with the cosmetic dentist, the patient may never be satisfied. The end result will not meet his/her expectations. And they will never know why.

Lips can also be crooked on one side of the midline of the face and normal on the other. When lips are higher on one side of the midline than on the other, the teeth on the side with the higher lip line will appear larger than the teeth on the other side because more tooth structure shows when the lip is higher (figure 10).

13

A very common lip variation is called a "high lip line," giving a patient a "gummy" smile (figure 11). This occurs when the muscles of the mouth pull the upper lip up too high when smiling or speaking, or when the bone supporting the upper teeth (maxillary bone) is too prominent. On most people's smiles, the lips cover the part of the teeth that enters the gum line (called the gingival margins). The actual gum line appearance in these patients is not cosmetically important because it can't be seen when smiling. When the lip line is high, the gums and shape of the gingival contours play a more critical role in how the teeth and smile look.

Ideally, all the gingival margins should be even, as if they were lined up against an imaginary line at the top of all the teeth. Unfortunately, gingival margins are often at different levels, giving teeth an unbalanced look or a sense of unevenness. Whether it is a single tooth or a group of teeth that have uneven gingival margins, it should be corrected if the gums show when the person smiles. Otherwise, eyes will always focus on the uneven gum line when the person smiles (figure 12). If the gums are covering too much tooth structure, correction can be accomplished by simple surgical procedures such as gingivectomies, crown lengthenings, and gum lifts.

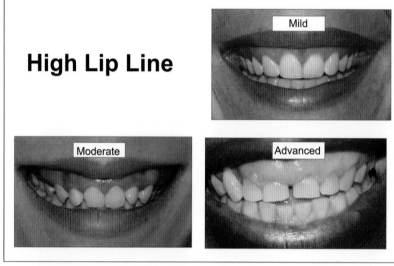

figure 11

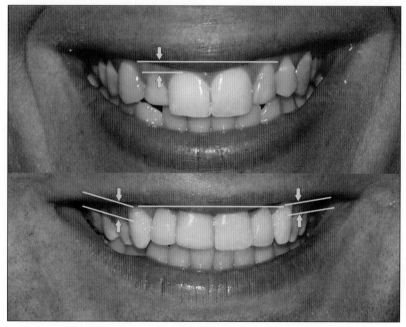

figure 12

Other times, the opposite problem exists and there is not enough gum tissue covering the teeth. The gum line appears much too high in the maxilla or too low in the mandible when the patient smiles. This gives the teeth a very long and unnatural look, and they seem out of balance with the others. If the problem is minimal, a piece of gum tissue can be grafted onto the elongated tooth root recreating a normal appearing tooth (figure 12b). If the gum line is extremely receded, or the patient is not a candidate for gum grafting (gingival grafts), more extensive restorative procedures are performed. For example, teeth can be restored using either porcelain veneers, crowns or fixed bridges, and pink porcelain can be added to these restorations to create the illusion of natural gum tissue. These types of restorations are particularly useful where teeth have been lost or gums have receded (figure 13).

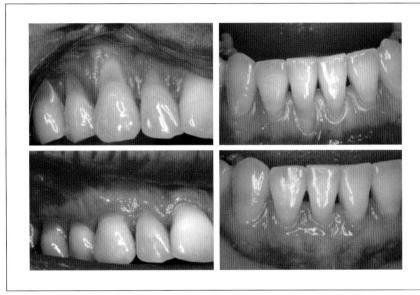

figure 12b

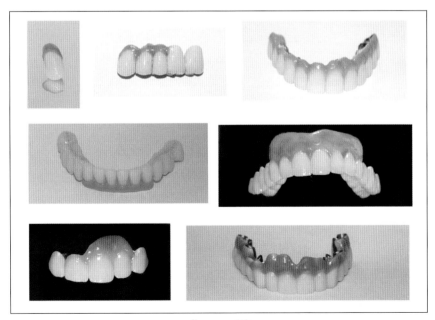

figure 13

As mentioned earlier, teeth are arranged on either the maxillary arch or the mandibular arch. The shapes of these arches can vary as well. The arch can be oval or rounded, square or tapered (figure 14). These individually shaped arches can also be wide, average or narrow.

The shape and width of the arch will affect how the teeth and smile look when viewed from the front of the face. Besides affecting the overall look of a smile, the width of the arches will particularly affect the appearance of the corners of the mouth. Looking closely at a smile, it is noticeable that the average smile has a slight triangular shadow between the posterior teeth and the corners of the mouth. This is called the buccal corridor. The buccal corridor is influenced by the size and shape of the arch form. These arch form variations can create completely different looks in the mouth. For example, in some mouths, the arch form is very wide creating a broad full smile and little buccal corridor. This creates a very "toothy" look or "wide smile" (figure15).

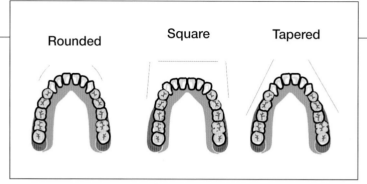

figure 14

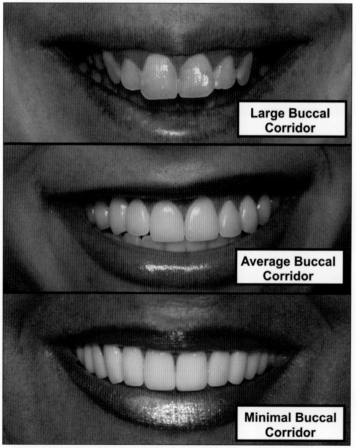

figure 15

16

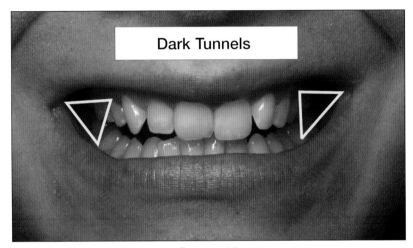

figure 16

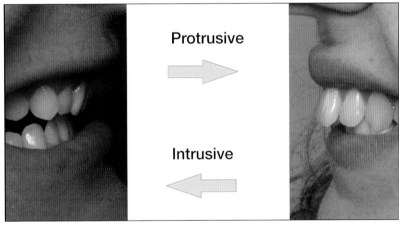

figure 17

In others, the arch may be tapered or narrow creating huge triangular shadows. This creates a situation where little if any posterior teeth can be seen, resulting in the illusion of huge dark tunnels when this person smiles (figure 16). These triangular shadows can be decreased by changing the arch form and width.

As we focus on the anterior teeth we see interesting tooth relationships between the maxillary and mandibular arches. When we examine the maxillary front teeth we notice that they can be in a normal relationship to the lower teeth, protrusive (too far forward) or intrusive (slanted in) (figure 17).

When anterior teeth overlap, this is referred to as an overbite. To be technically correct, specific names are used when referring to overbite variations. When looking at a person's smile from the side, the protrusion of the maxillary incisors beyond the edges of the mandibular incisors on a horizontal plane is called the overjet. The amount that the maxillary incisors hang vertically down over the mandibular incisors is called the overbite (figure 18).

These terms are often confusing. You can have an overjet with or without an overbite. Or you can have a deep overbite with great or little overjet.

Looking at the teeth from the frontal view, the six maxillary teeth have the greatest influence on the look of a smile. Therefore, special attention must be given to how the maxillary anterior teeth look and how they are arranged.

Anterior teeth come in many shapes and sizes. Teeth can be square, tapered or ovoid. There can also be a combination of these shapes, such as square tapered or square ovoid (figure 19). Several combinations of tooth shapes can be used within an arch. A person can choose ovoid incisors and pointed canines. Or they can choose square and flat incisors and rounded canines. This is part of the artistic creative process that makes a particular smile unique and attractive.

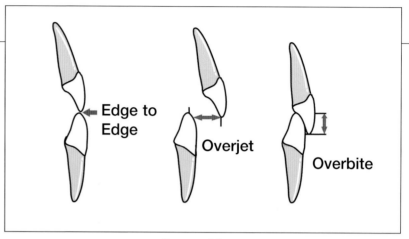

figure 18

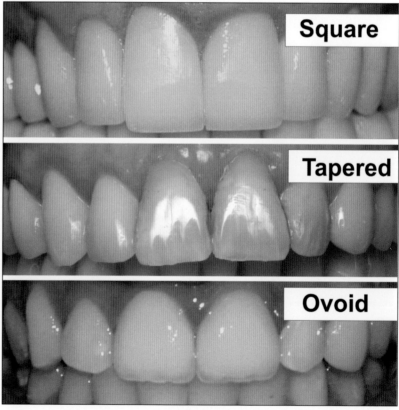

figure 19

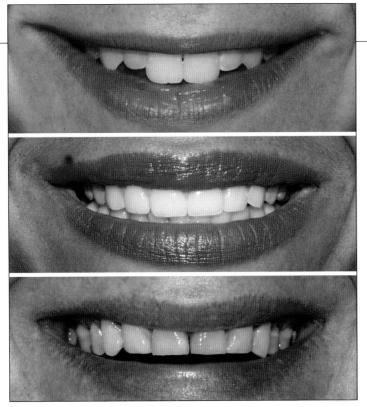

figure 20

Once the correct shape is selected, the focus should shift to how the teeth line up on a straight line (the horizontal plane), as viewed from the front of the patient (figure 20). Remember, this horizontal plane should be parallel to the inter-pupillary line that connects the center of both eyes. There are many variations at the edges of the teeth, in relation to this line. The edges of the maxillary teeth (the incisal edges) may line up on a straight line, or they may be arranged so that the maxillary lateral incisors are shorter to varying degrees than the central incisors. Staggered incisal edges make a smile appear more natural and more youthful. Incisal edges on a flat plane make the edges look more worn. Worn edges are more commonly found in patients who grind their teeth or older patients as they wear down their teeth over time.

Color is another important consideration in the smile design process. There are dozens of tooth colors available. Generally speaking, it should be discussed with the cosmetic dentist whether a white smile look or a "natural" look is preferred. Teeth naturally are not very white, but have more cream-like or light yellow overtones. The specific colors of individual teeth can be chosen from shade ranges on dental shade guides. A cosmetic dentist can provide many shade guides from which to choose (figure 21). For a more natural look, different color shades may be used within the same arch. For example, canines are naturally darker than incisors or posterior teeth.

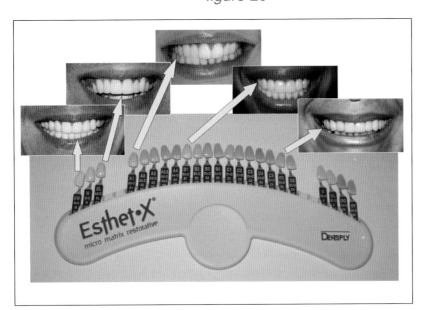

figure 21

Choosing the correct color of teeth can be tricky. Given the same size teeth, the lighter the teeth are, the larger they will look. If teeth are more pronounced and forward in the arch form because of an individual's specific anatomy, very light colored teeth should not be chosen. They will not look attractive. Instead, the color should be toned down (figure21b). Similarly, when teeth are naturally very large or very long, very white colors should be avoided. On the contrary, if teeth are small or recessed in the mouth, lighter colored teeth will make the smile look better.

If only select teeth are being restored, it is important that the color chosen for these teeth blend in with the remaining teeth in the arch. This color does not necessarily have to be a perfect match if the other teeth don't really show when smiling. However, they should be in the same range of color. If you are choosing to change the look of your front teeth, color will influence the complexity of your smile makeover. The lighter the color selected, the more teeth will have to be restored for the resulting smile to look natural and attractive. The average smile makeover requires a minimum of eight to ten maxillary teeth to be cosmetically improved in order to attain a great looking smile. If the lower teeth show when you smile, six to eight mandibular teeth may also have to be restored to compliment the look of the new maxillary teeth. If minimal mandibular teeth show when you smile, it may be enough to just bleach your lower teeth to make them brighter (figure 21c).

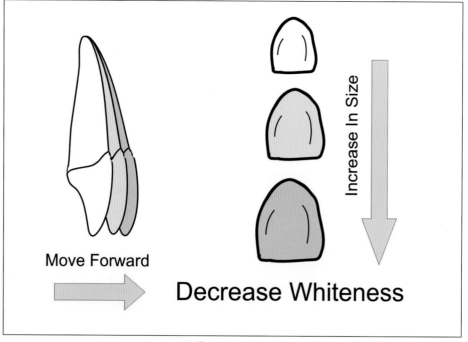

figure 21b

Mandibular Smile Teeth

Requires 4-6 veneers

Requires 8-10 veneers

Requires all lower veneers

figure 21c

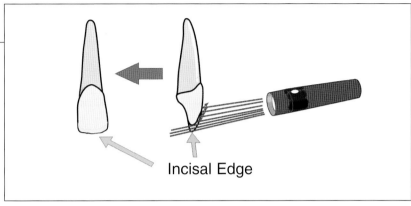

figure 22

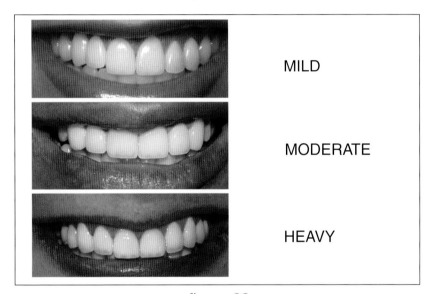

figure 23

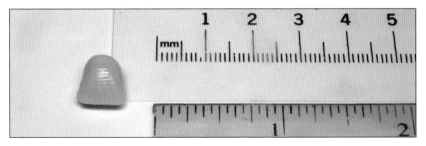

figure 24

In addition to the colors, shapes, sizes and arrangements of teeth, the patient and the cosmetic dentist must also consider the biting edges of the anterior teeth. These biting edges, called the incisal edges, have a different property of enamel than the remaining tooth structure (figure 22).

At the incisal edge, the enamel is usually more translucent than the thin enamel covering the the body of the tooth. This translucency allows light to easily pass through the incisal edge, giving the edge a blue-gray look.

This blue-gray look is caused by the backdrop and shadowing of the deepest part of the mouth showing through the translucent enamel. It should be decided by the cosmetic dentist and the patient if a mild, moderate or heavy amount of translucency is preferred (figure 23).

Another important fact to be aware of is how cosmetic dentists measure teeth. They measure tooth size in millimeters, not inches. Don't refer to the customary inch scale when asking to have teeth lengthened, widened or changed. Millimeters may be very tiny, but adding just a millimeter can have a dramatic visual effect upon teeth and smiles (figure 24).

Finally, no discussion about cosmetic dentistry would be complete without mentioning the "golden proportion". The golden proportion was identified during the time of ancient Greece. When visualizing many objects in nature, it was discovered that there seemed to be a logical relationship or constant proportion between those objects that could be measured. Interestingly, in mathematics and science, those same proportions could be found over and over again (figure 25).

The golden proportion is a measurable and repetitious pattern that is found throughout nature. When objects contain this golden proportion they are usually visually appealing. When two objects are in the golden proportion the larger object is 1.618 times the size of the smaller object. This relationship is measurable by a "golden proportion gauge" (figure 25).

This formula can be seen in all of biology and throughout nature. Since it was discovered, it has been used by architects and designers throughout the ages (figure 25b).

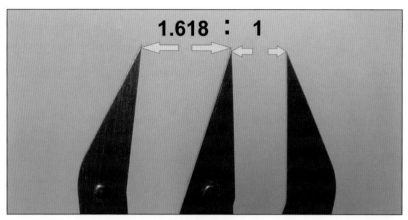

figure 25

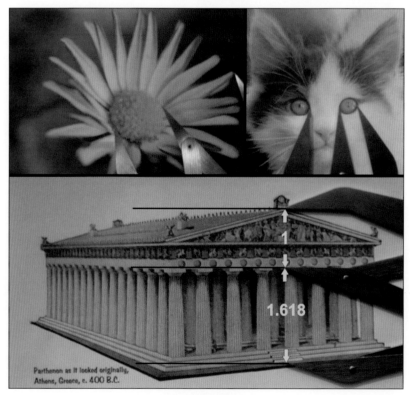

figure 25b

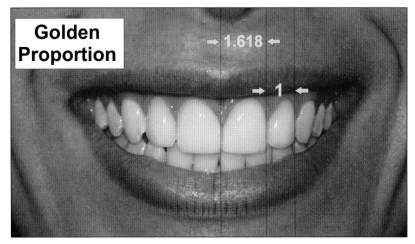

figure 26

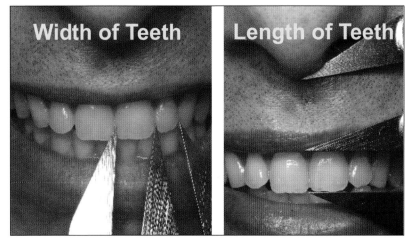

figure 26b

When teeth are arranged within the golden proportion, they appear visually attractive. Teeth are arranged in the golden proportion to each other as well as to other landmarks on the face. Figure 26 demonstrates how teeth are in a golden proportion to each other and how the length of teeth are in a golden proportion to the length of the upper lip (figure 26b).

The golden proportion should be used as a guiding principle when creating aesthetically beautiful teeth.

A basic understanding of dental anatomy will go a long way in effectively opening the channels of communication between patient and cosmetic dentist. A little knowledge of dental basics and guidelines allows patients to become a part of the creative process.

COSMETIC DENTAL PROCEDURES

Various dental materials are used during cosmetic dental procedures to restore and replace teeth. These materials, along with the way they are used, have a profound effect on the way a smile ultimately looks. When dentists started using a material known as composite resin, more commonly known as bonding, the first dramatic cosmetic changes were seen. This material brought modern cosmetic dentistry into the forefront of today's dental care. Bonding is used in a putty or liquid form to cover, repair, extend or replace tooth surfaces (figure 27).

The tooth receiving the bonding material is etched with a mild acid, making it more porous. The bonding composite resin is applied, fused and hardened with a light gun. Finally, the bonded material is shaped, adjusted and polished. Bonded, composite resins are excellent materials for filling small caries (cavities), and for repairs at the gum line. Bonding can also close small gaps between teeth. However, it does not hold up well when used to fill large holes on biting surfaces or on the incisal edges of teeth.

The first real public awareness of cosmetic dentistry occurred when cosmetic dentists began performing complete smile makeovers. These early pioneers in cosmetic dentistry changed or replaced

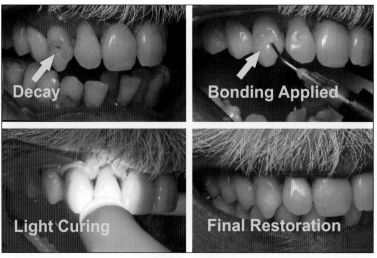

figure 27

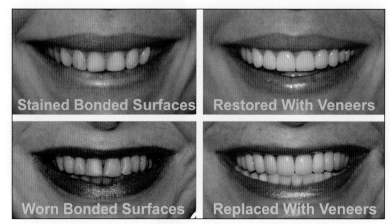

figure 28

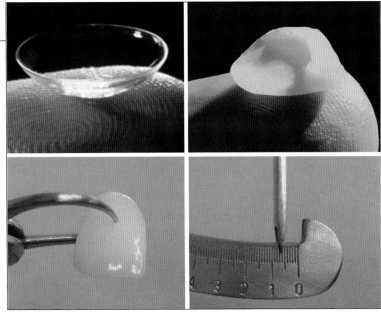

figure 29

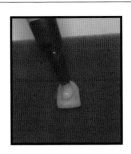

Adhesive applied to veneer

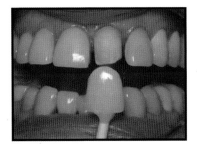

Veneer being placed on prepared tooth

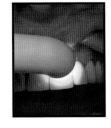

Curing veneer to tooth with light.

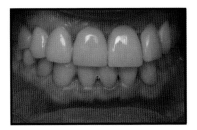

Final veneer in place

figure 30

the entire outer surfaces of the anterior teeth with bonded composite resins. This changed the way teeth looked when the patient smiled. Although the results were dramatic, many times the bonded material for full smile makeovers did not withstand the test of time. Often, the bonded surfaces would break or wear down. Other times, they would absorb stains which led to discoloration (figure 28).

A stronger and more permanent material had to be developed; hence, the porcelain veneer was created. Porcelain veneers are very thin pieces of porcelain (they can be made as thin as a contact lens), which fit directly over the outside of existing teeth (figure 29). They are permanently fused to existing tooth structure with a liquified bonding adhesive which is cured by a special curing light (figure 30).

In order to avoid creating teeth that look too bulky, (caused by layering too much material on top of the teeth), a small amount of tooth structure must be removed. Doing so makes the final result look and feel more natural.

There is much publicity about drill-less thin veneers today. However, experience shows that this application has limitations. Most patients requiring porcelain veneers need some tooth reduction to obtain a natural and realistic result.

When teeth do not have enough natural tooth structure to support a porcelain veneer, a crown (cap) must be fabricated. The entire tooth surface must be removed with a dental drill so that a full tooth covering can be made (figure 31).

There are several techniques for fabricating crowns. One type of crown has a metallic core which is covered by a thin layer of porcelain. It is held in place by dental cement. This is called a "porcelain-fused-to-metal crown" (figure 31b). When the inner core is gold, it is called a "porcelain-fused-to-gold crown." When porcelain-fused-to-metal or porcelain-fused-to-gold crowns are used, the metal inside the crown must be covered with an opaque layer to prevent the metal color from showing through the translucent porcelain. However, opaque layers affect the color quality of these types of crowns. They often look too harsh or "dead" because of their poor reflective qualities and lack of translucency. This effect can be improved by using a high carat alloy gold inside the crown. In addition, careful staining by a very talented dental technician can sometimes overcome this opaque look to make the crown look more natural. However, this is not an easy task and it truly involves a great deal of talent and experience.

If the crown cannot be seen when smiling, it can be made entirely of metal, such as gold. However, for the purpose of this book, we will concentrate on cosmetically visible crowns, as their aesthetic requirements are different.

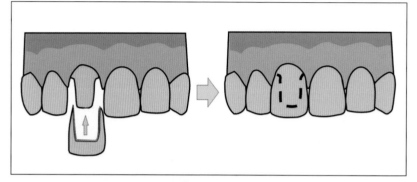

figure 31

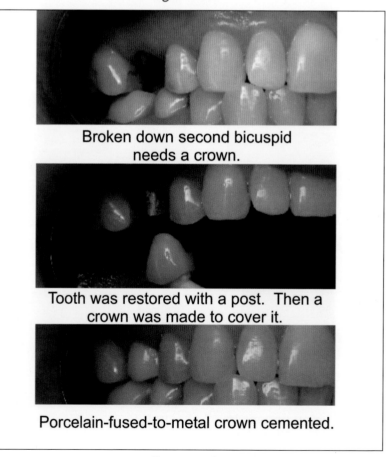

Broken down second bicuspid needs a crown.

Tooth was restored with a post. Then a crown was made to cover it.

Porcelain-fused-to-metal crown cemented.

figure 31b

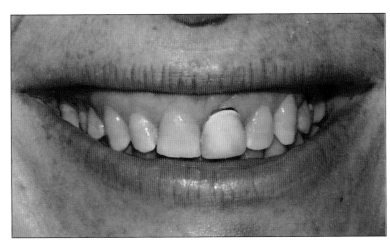

figure 32

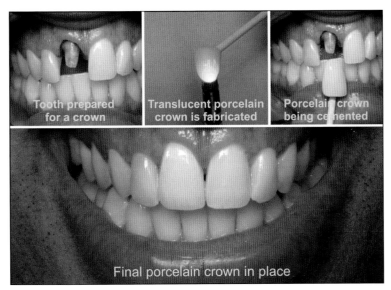

Tooth prepared for a crown

Translucent porcelain crown is fabricated

Porcelain crown being cemented

Final porcelain crown in place

figure 33

Another problem associated with porcelain-fused-to-metal crowns is the black line phenomenon (figure 32). The black line appears because the porcelain-fused-to-metal crown must end at or below the gum line with an all-metal margin. Dentists usually try to hide this black line by preparing the tooth deep enough below the gum line so that the metal margin does not show. However, many patient's gums are thin and translucent and the dark line shows through. Some patients have gum recession over time, exposing the black line of the metal margin, which originally did not show. The "black line" phenomenon is eliminated when using an "all porcelain crown" (figure 33).

The greatest advantage of all porcelain crowns is that they look more natural in the mouth. This is due to the fact that, similar to a natural tooth, light transmits through the porcelain.

As mentioned earlier, bonded, composite restorations were the first cosmetic restorations performed in modern cosmetic dentistry. They are routinely used to add contour to teeth, to correct small spaces, or to fill small cavities caused by decay. Sometimes, the hole left in the tooth by decay is very large. Other times, large, dark, gray, old silver fillings must be replaced. The resulting holes left on these teeth are much too large for bonded, composite restorations. The bonded, composite restorations are simply not strong enough to withstand the chewing forces to which the teeth will be subjected. Yet there is enough healthy tooth structure left so that a full crown does not have to be placed on the tooth. The restoration of choice for this situation is the "inlay."

Originally, inlays were fabricated from solid gold. However, our cosmetically conscious society demanded more attractive restorations. The result was the development of the composite inlay, the porcelain inlay, and porcelain-fused-to-gold inlay. Porcelain inlays, although attractive, have a high fracture rate. Composite inlays are more resilient and are commonly used today. They are fabricated in the dental lab out of a very aesthetic tooth-colored material. Once sent back to the dentist they are permanently cemented into large cavities prepared in teeth, providing strong and lifelike restorations that can last several decades (figure 34).

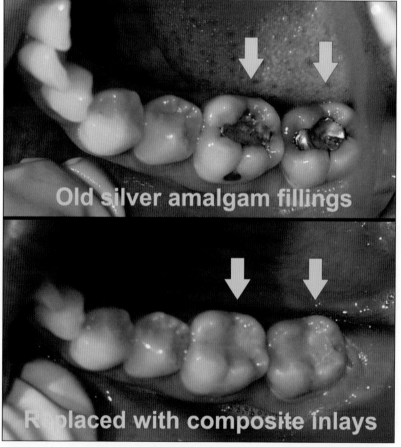

Old silver amalgam fillings

Replaced with composite inlays

figure 34

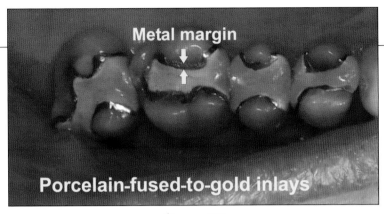

figure 35

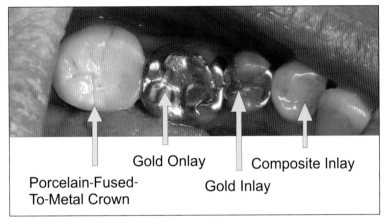

Porcelain-Fused-
To-Metal Crown

Gold Onlay

Gold Inlay

Composite Inlay

figure 35b

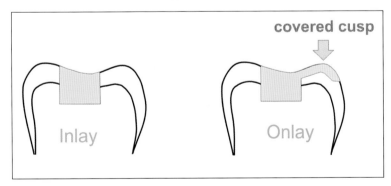

figure 36

A much stronger and more enduring restoration is the "porcelain-fused-to-gold" inlay (figure 35). These inlays have the advantage of the strength of metal with the aesthetic covering of porcelain. However, the aesthetics are compromised because the tiny metal margin can be seen, and the opaque liner on top of the metal distorts the shade of the porcelain. These restorations are most suitable for the back part of the mouth, where they often do not compromise a patient's smile.

If the restoration cannot be seen when the patient smiles, the gold inlay is still the standard by which all filling materials are compared (figure 35b). Gold inlays, when properly made, can last the lifetime of the patient, provided the patient maintains his or her mouth properly. As new porcelain technology develops and more durable cements are created, porcelain inlays may approach the gold inlay for long lasting durability and function. One final note; if an inlay is large enough to cover a cusp of a tooth (the bumps on top of teeth) it is referred to as an onlay rather than an inlay (figure 36).

The greatest cosmetic challenge occurs when teeth are missing from the mouth. When one or more teeth are missing, there are several options to consider. These options range from removable appliances called dentures or partial dentures, to fixed bridges, to dental implants.

If there is sufficient bone where a tooth is missing, a dental implant is the restoration of choice (figure 37). Dental implants are metallic cylinders (like a wide screw) that are placed directly into the bone where the lost tooth root once existed. The implant fuses to the surrounding bone by a process called osseointegration. This process can take from four to six months. When the implant finally osseointegrates, a post (called an abutment) is placed into the dental implant. A crown is then placed on top of the implant, permanently replacing the missing tooth (figure 38).

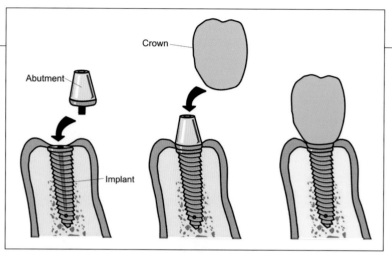

figure 37

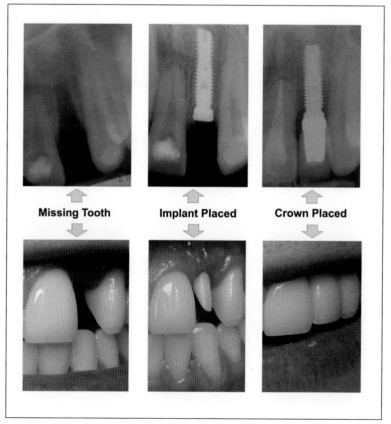

figure 38

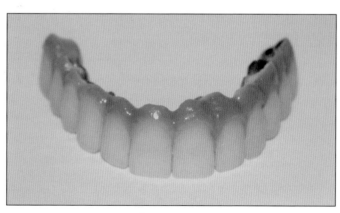

figure 38b

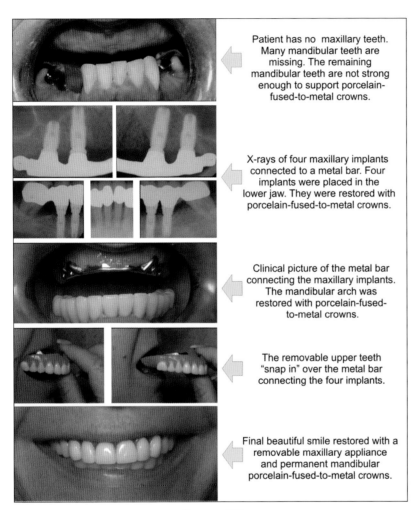

Patient has no maxillary teeth. Many mandibular teeth are missing. The remaining mandibular teeth are not strong enough to support porcelain-fused-to-metal crowns.

X-rays of four maxillary implants connected to a metal bar. Four implants were placed in the lower jaw. They were restored with porcelain-fused-to-metal crowns.

Clinical picture of the metal bar connecting the maxillary implants. The mandibular arch was restored with porcelain-fused-to-metal crowns.

The removable upper teeth "snap in" over the metal bar connecting the four implants.

Final beautiful smile restored with a removable maxillary appliance and permanent mandibular porcelain-fused-to-metal crowns.

figure 39

When all teeth are missing in one arch, the patient may choose to have them replaced with multiple dental implants. There are many ways to restore teeth over dental implants. Deciding factors include the amount of available bone for implantation and the costs associated with restoring the actual teeth. If enough bone is available, porcelain or porcelain-fused-to-metal crowns over the implant abutment will provide the most natural looking results (figure 38b).

A less costly alternative might be plastic teeth fused to a metal framework, which is then secured to the implants below. Either way, these restorations are permanent and not removable by the patient.

If only a limited amount of bone is available after the loss of all the teeth in one arch, only two or four implants are usually placed. Upon these implants, a metallic bar can be fastened. Then a full set of teeth will be fabricated that can "clip" or "snap" onto the bar, thereby holding the teeth in place (figure 39). This is called a fitted removable prosthesis or an overdenture.

There are times when not enough bone is available. Other times, medical conditions, or financial considerations may preclude tooth replacement with dental implants.

If teeth exist on either side of the space created by the lost teeth, another solution is a fixed bridge (figure 40).

A fixed bridge consists of preparing the teeth and placing a crown on either side of the space created by the missing tooth/teeth. An impression of the prepared teeth is taken and sent to a dental lab. At the lab, a model of the mouth with the prepared teeth is made. The technician will make two crowns, one for each prepared tooth on either side of the space. A fake dummy tooth (called a pontic) is fused to the two fabricated crowns, thus creating a fixed bridge. The entire fixed bridge (two crowns and pontic) is sent back to the dentist and is permanently cemented onto the two prepared teeth in the patient's mouth. The missing tooth is now replaced.

Fixed bridges, like crowns, can be made of porcelain-fused-to-gold, porcelain-fused-to-metal, or all porcelain. The same considerations for cosmetics and the rules for strength apply as they do for crowns (figure 41).

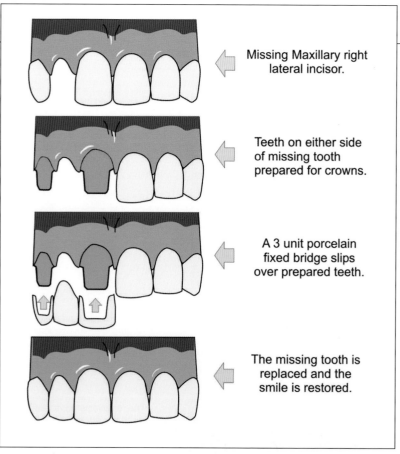

Missing Maxillary right lateral incisor.

Teeth on either side of missing tooth prepared for crowns.

A 3 unit porcelain fixed bridge slips over prepared teeth.

The missing tooth is replaced and the smile is restored.

figure 40

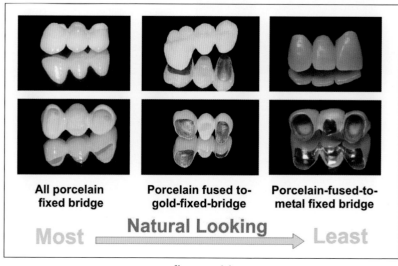

| All porcelain fixed bridge | Porcelain fused to-gold-fixed-bridge | Porcelain-fused-to-metal fixed bridge |

Natural Looking

Most ⟶ Least

figure 41

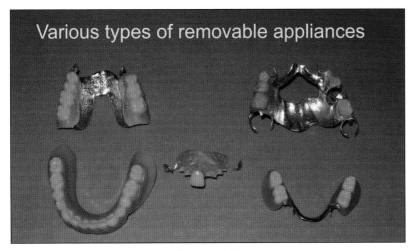

figure 42

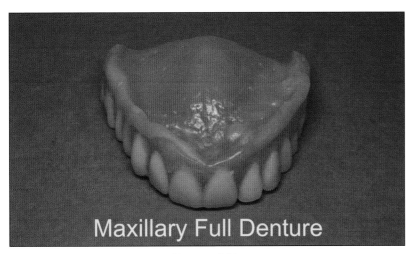

figure 42b

Sometimes many teeth or all teeth are missing. Fixed bridges or implants may not be options due to lack of quality or quantity of available bone. In these cases, partial or full dentures may be the only option.

Partial dentures are used when there are a few remaining teeth available to attach to an appliance. The attachments can be made of metallic clasps or invisible semi-precision attachments (figure 42). The attachments stabilize the partial denture during eating.

Dentures are made when all the teeth are missing in one arch (figure 42b). Fit and comfort depends on the amount of available bone and the quantity and quality of the patient's saliva.

Although partial dentures and full dentures provide aesthetic replacement of teeth, they often lack in function and chewing efficiency. These appliances are also removable. Many patients, psychologically, cannot bear the idea of removing their teeth nightly to clean them or to give their remaining teeth and gums a rest. Sometimes, however, the situation is such that this remains the only choice for the patient. Full dentures and partial dentures are considerably less expensive than fixed bridges and dental implants. Financial considerations are a reality and dentures are a viable alternative. Once again, the talent and experience of the cosmetic dentist will play a role in both alleviating the concerns of the patient, and getting the best result functionally and aesthetically.

For many patients, teeth do not always have to be replaced or restored. They just may need to be lightened and brightened in order to look better. The solution is often teeth bleaching. There are many over-the-counter bleaching products available that have some limited ability to whiten teeth. For the most efficacious and safest way to bleach your teeth, you should consider professionally administered tooth whitening by your cosmetic dentist.

There are two ways to professionally bleach and lighten your teeth. One method is with an in-office bleaching system that requires about an hour of your time (figure 43). Once your teeth are isolated, a strong bleaching agent is applied. Your teeth are then placed under a powerful light source that activates the bleaching agent. Your teeth will be brighter in about one hour.

A second technique for bleaching your teeth is performed by creating a thin, soft, custom tray that fits over your teeth. This is called a 'bleaching tray' (figure 44). A bleaching gel is placed inside the tray by the patient. It is worn in the mouth at home for a few hours each day or night. The maximum benefit from this technique will be seen in four to six weeks.

Whether an in-office bleaching technique, or an in-home bleaching tray technique is used, all teeth bleaching tends to fade over time.

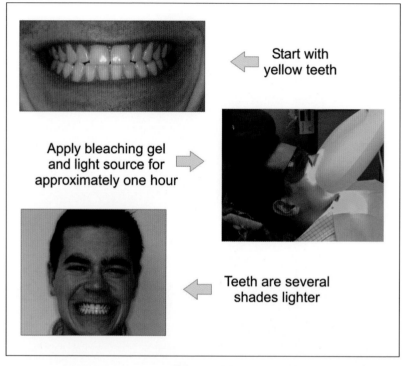

figure 43

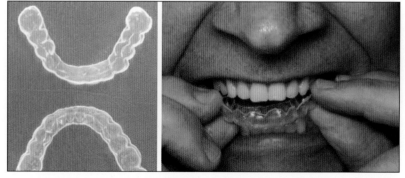

figure 44

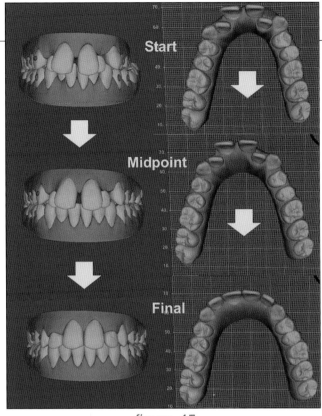

figure 45

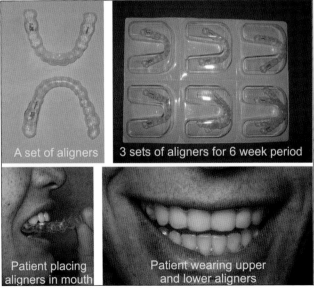

figure 46

You should use custom bleaching trays every few months at home to restore faded brightness.

If a patient has healthy and beautiful teeth, but they just need them straightened, a good way to achieve this cosmetically is with Invisalign® aligners. Invisalign® is an orthodontic treatment method using invisible or clear trays called aligners, that fit snuggly over your teeth. The technique is simple and very accurate. To correct mal-aligned teeth, an impression is taken of the teeth and sent to the Invisalign® laboratory. At the lab, the impression is scanned into a computer. On the computer, the software program calculates how to straighten the teeth, how long it will take, and how to design the aligners (figure 45).

Once the aligners are fabricated they are returned to the dentist. The dentist will give the patient three sets of aligners. Each set is worn for two weeks (figure 46).

The aligners are worn by the patient about 20 hours per day. The patient has to return to the dentist to check the tooth movement every six weeks.

Aligners do not interfere with speech and are very comfortable to wear. They are virtually invisible. Results are often very dramatic (figure 47 and 47b).

Invisalign® tooth movement and correction can take anywhere from six months for simple cases, to 18 months or longer for more complex cases. It is truly the most conservative way to move and straighten teeth.

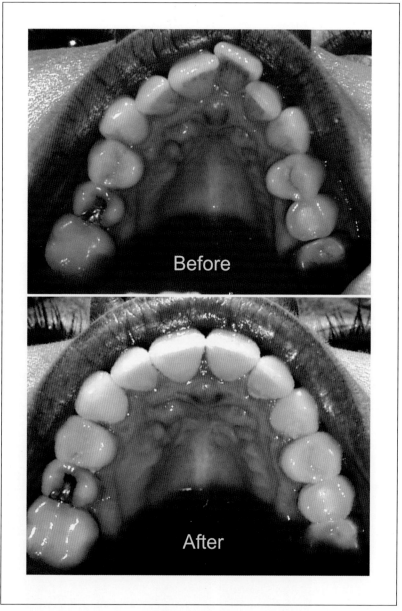

figure 47b

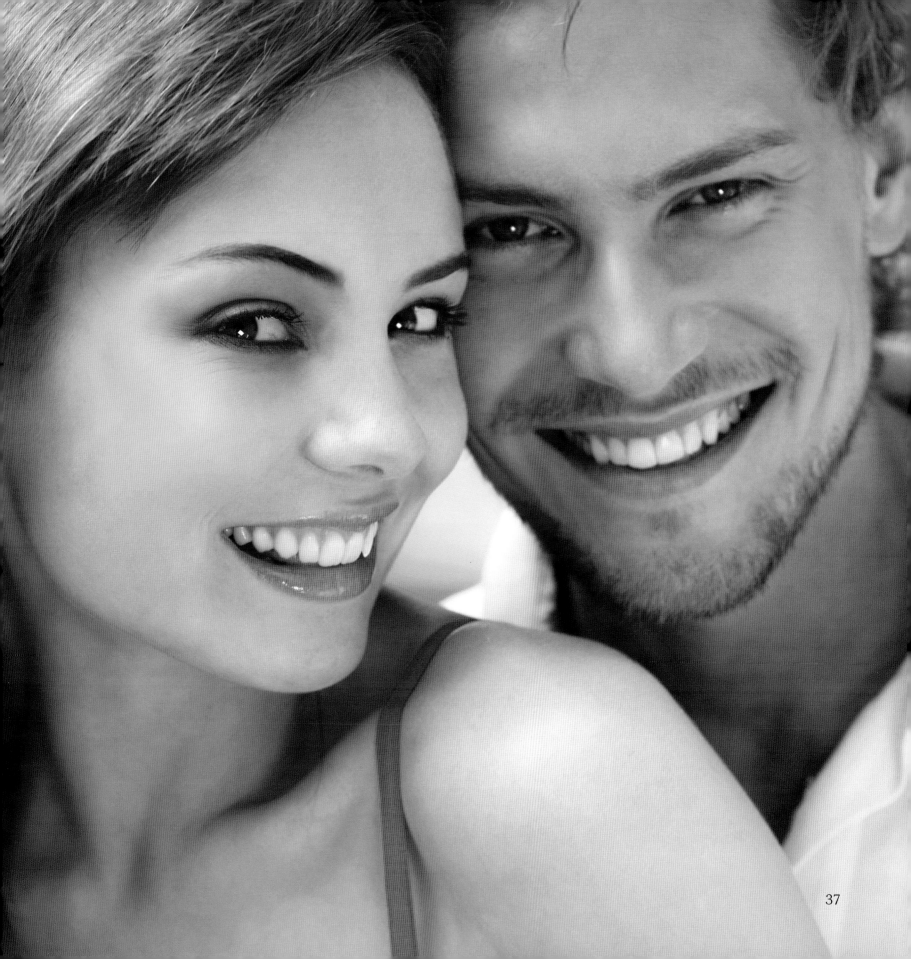

Miracles in Two Visits:
The Porcelain Veneer

Since the majority of smile makeovers today involve porcelain veneers, this revolutionary procedure warrants special attention. Although porcelain veneers (porcelain laminates) have been around since the 1980s, their popularity did not materialize until years later. A series of cosmetic makeover television shows and news reports revealed the benefits and showcased the dramatic differences they made. The results from smile makeovers with porcelain veneers are always astounding and amazing.

What makes porcelain veneers so attractive is two-fold:

1) they can dramatically change a smile in as little as two dental visits; and

2) the procedure is virtually painless.

Even the most fearful patient can comfortably have a new smile in a short period of time with porcelain veneers. As mentioned in chapter three, porcelain veneers are thin eggshell-like pieces of porcelain that can be made in any color, shape or size. They are only about one millimeter or less in thickness (figure 48).

In order to receive veneers, the teeth need to be decay free with a minimal thickness of enamel

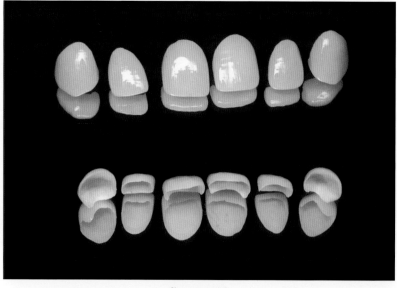

figure 48

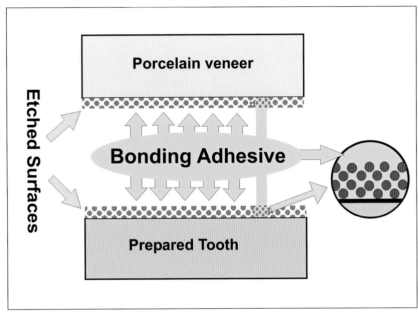

figure 49

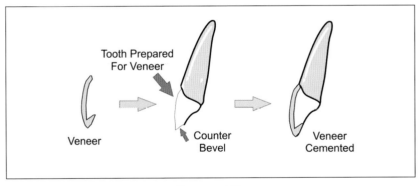

figure 49b

present. The reason enamel is needed, even after some minor tooth reduction, is because the porcelain veneer adheres to the tooth through its enamel.

When porcelain veneers come back from the dental lab, they are highly glazed on the outside. The inside (the side that will be adhering to the tooth) is micro-porous and frosty looking. This frosty appearance was created by application of an acid at the dental lab.

The cosmetic dentist will use a safe, milder acid in the mouth to quickly etch the remaining enamel on the prepared tooth to receive the veneer. Once etched, the tooth surface has micropores; with both surfaces etched (figure 49), a liquid composite resin is used to cement the etched veneer to the etched tooth.

If not enough enamel is present on the tooth, or not enough tooth structure is available, the porcelain veneer will not adhere to the tooth, and may fall off during function. In order to add additional strength and stability to porcelain veneers, the teeth are prepared over the incisal edges and wrapped onto the lingual surfaces. This process is known as a counter bevel (figure 49b).

Here is an actual case study of a typical porcelain veneer smile makeover.

This patient has unsightly maxillary teeth. Her objective is to eliminate the spaces between her teeth and get rid of the "gummy" smile look (figure 50).

After administration of local anesthetic, her maxillary gums and bone are reduced and allowed to heal for six weeks (figure 51).

Once the gums are healed, the eight maxillary teeth are prepared for porcelain veneers (figure 52).

A dental impression of the prepared teeth is taken and sent to the lab. Temporary bonded veneers are made for the patient to wear for one week (figure 53).

In the lab, the ceramist makes the individual veneers by hand, carefully coloring each one to simulate natural tooth structure. They are then fired in a porcelain oven at over 2000 degrees Fahrenheit until they turn into a glasslike substance. They are now ready to be returned to the cosmetic dentist (figure 54).

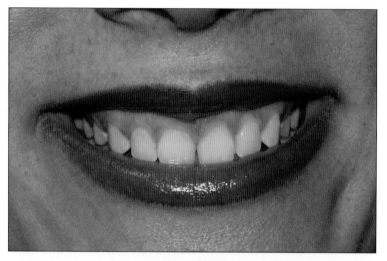

figure 50

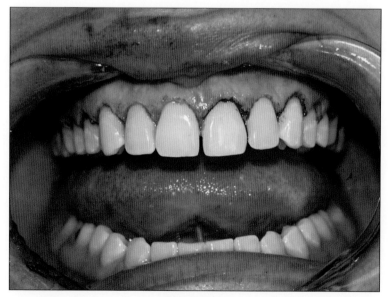

figure 51

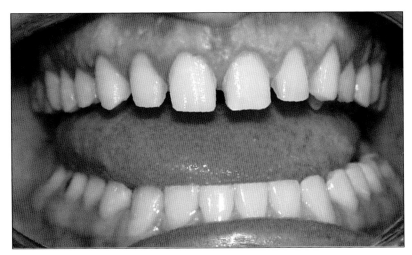

figure 52

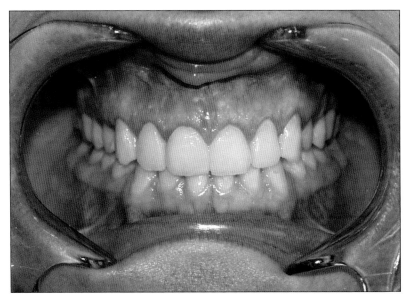

figure 53

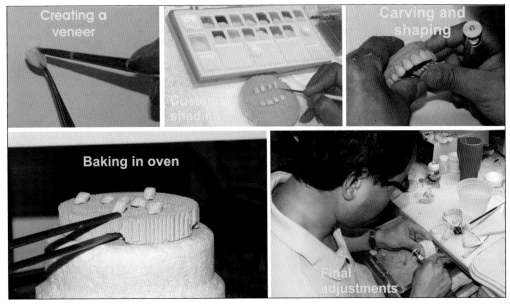

figure 54

Upon receipt of the veneers, the cosmetic dentist tries the veneers on the prepared teeth to check the fitting and get the patient's aesthetic approval. This is the patient's final opportunity to make changes. At this point the veneers can still be sent back to the lab for corrections (figure 55).

Once approved by the patient, the cosmetic dentist etches each tooth with a mild acid (figure 56). The dentist then applies a bonding adhesive to the inside of each porcelain veneer (figure 56b).

The veneer is placed on the etched tooth and cured with a high wavelength curing light for several seconds (figure 57).

The excess adhesive is removed and the bite (occlusion) is adjusted. The final veneers are now complete. The spaces are eliminated and the "gummy smile" look is gone. The smile makeover is brought to a successful conclusion (figure 58).

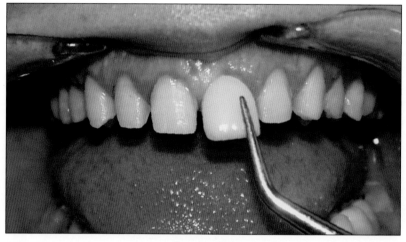

figure 56

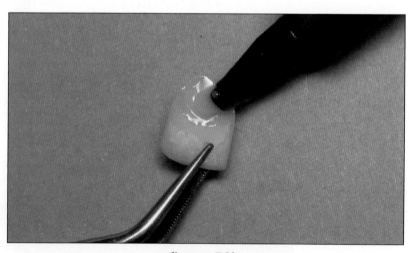

figure 56b

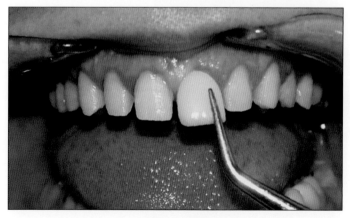

figure 55

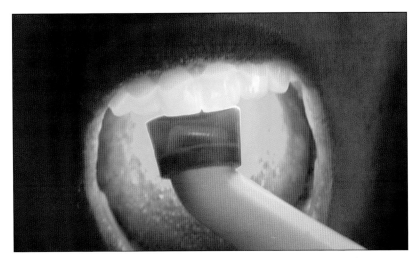

figure 57

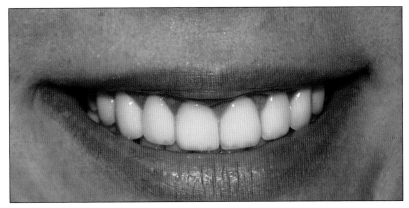

figure 58

TRY BEFORE YOU BUY - WHAT WILL MY SMILE LOOK LIKE?

Many times the anticipated change in one's smile may create a level of anxiety for the patient. At the same time, the expectations of the patient may be unclearly defined, creating concern for the cosmetic dentist. They both need to know in a very general way, what the final result will look like. Unfortunately, many smile makeover procedures with ceramic material, especially porcelain veneers, cannot be temporarily placed in the mouth on a trial basis. Once they are made in the lab, and verified in the mouth, they must be permanently cemented. There is no way to temporarily cement the thin ceramic material to the prepared tooth without it breaking or immediately falling off.

Sometimes, an approximate preview of the final result is necessary before the smile makeover can proceed.

There are three options to preview a smile, all having certain limitations. The first is called cosmetic imaging. Your cosmetic dentist can take a pre-operative digital photograph of your smile and perform cosmetic imaging on a computer, to simulate how your new smile might look (figure 59).

The nice thing about imaging is that it is quick and easy for the cosmetic dentist to do. If

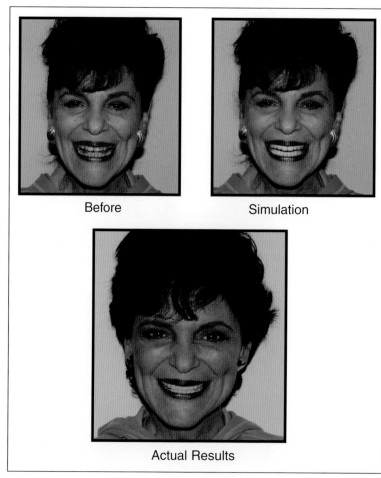

Before

Simulation

Actual Results

figure 59

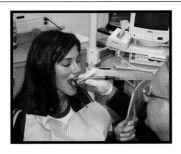

Cosmetic dentist creating "mock up" in the mouth with bonding, to show the patient a suggested increase in length of her anterior teeth.

Now the patient compares different lengths of teeth on one side of her mouth against her original teeth length on the other side.

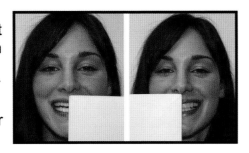

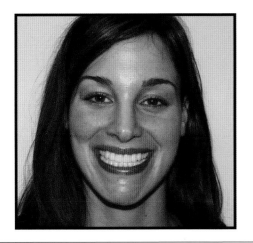

Final porcelain veneers are created to the desired length requested and approved by the patient.

figure 60

you don't like something, just change it. Teeth can be made to look longer, shorter, wider or whiter to name just a few variations. Unfortunately, you can do things on the computer that cannot actually be reproduced in the mouth. That is why many cosmetic imaging preview pictures look different than the final results. Cosmetic imaging on a computer can be used as a practical guide as long as the patient understands that the final results may and do vary.

A second alternative way to preview a smile is called a mock-up, made with composite bonding materials. With a mock-up, composite bonding materials are applied onto the unprepared teeth. Possible changes in the mouth are created for the patient to see. The cosmetic procedures are limited by the fact that no tooth structure is removed. The result may appear "bulkier" than the final result. As long as the patient understands this fact, the technique has a lot of merit. Another limitation is the cosmetic dentist. He/she may not have the artistic ability to create the desired result with composite. If the individual dentist lacks this talent or ability this technique should not be used.

When the mock-up guide is acceptable to the patient, an impression of it is taken and a duplicate stone cast made, which is then sent to the ceramist. This will be used as a guide for the final restoration. This technique is particularly useful when teeth are to be made larger or longer or the arch form needs to be built out for a wider smile appearance (figure 60).

Sometimes the bite relationship must be changed to achieve an acceptable cosmetic result.

This is particularly true when the bite must be opened to correct a cross bite situation (when the maxillary teeth are inside upon closing instead of overlapping outside the mandibular teeth). For this situation a laboratory can fabricate a temporary set of plastic like teeth with an open bite, called "snap on smile". This can be worn for a short period of time to see if the patient can tolerate the bite alteration. The advantage of the snap on smile is that it is removable. It can be brought home to show other people who might influence a patient's decisions about changing their smile. The disadvantage is that since they snap over the teeth and are made of a rubbery plastic, the results are often fake looking and bulky. This technique can be used as a guide when considering major changes to a smile. It can also be used when a patient needs a period of time to adjust to the new look (figure 61).

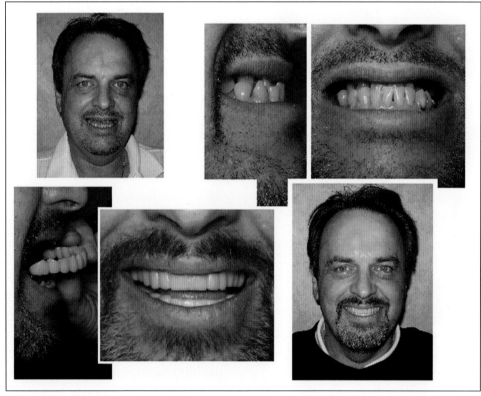

figure 61

The Smile Gallery
How Cosmetic Dentistry Can Change Your Smile

Now that you have a basic understanding of cosmetic dentistry, its language and terms, and the various procedures that make it all possible, it is time to see actual results in the smile gallery.

One thing is for sure... the results are always a dramatic improvement in the way a patient looks. So, go ahead and enjoy the smile gallery and see how these patients have improved their smiles and their lives through cosmetic dentistry.

DIASTEMA

This young woman presented with a "diastema", or space between her maxillary two central incisors. She also wanted to permanently brighten her overall smile.

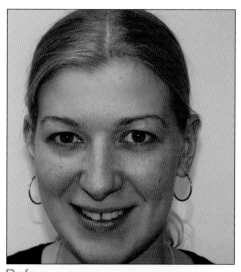

Before

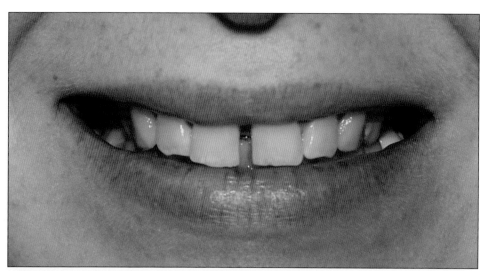

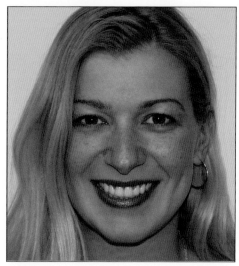

After

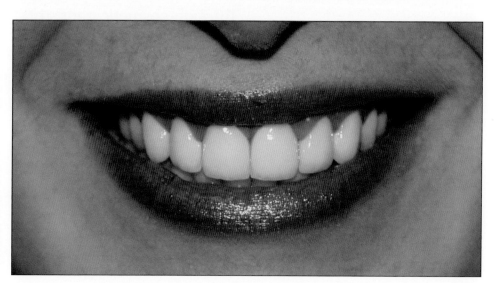

The solution was creating ten porcelain veneers which were applied to her maxillary teeth in just two easy visits. No more diastema and a brighter smile changed her entire facial look.

INTRUDED CENTRAL INCISORS

This patient was unhappy with her maxillary incisors. Her central incisors slanted in while her lateral incisors flared out. Too much gum tissue added an additional visual complication. Her bicuspid teeth slanted inward, creating a narrow arch.

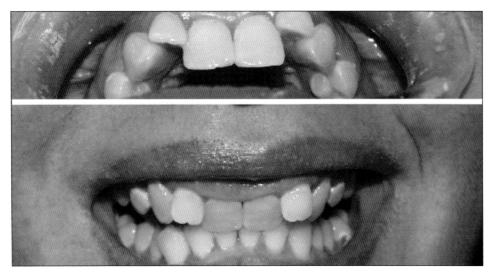

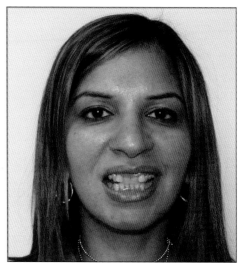

Before

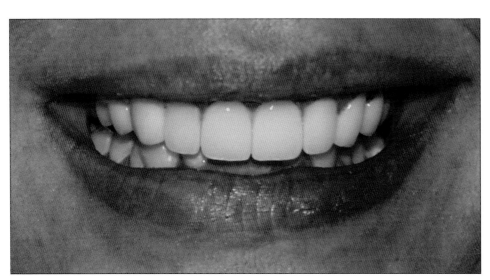

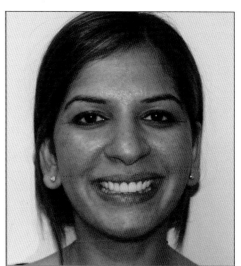

After

Her concerns were satisfied by trimming away the excess gum tissue above her maxillary central incisors and placing ten porcelain veneers. Her central incisors were brought forward while her lateral incisors were brought in. The outer surfaces of her bicuspids were brought out to broaden her arch. All this was accomplished in just two visits.

FLARED MAXILLARY INCISORS WITH SPACES

This patient was unhappy with her maxillary incisors flaring out. As the teeth moved forward, the spaces between them became more evident and unsightly.

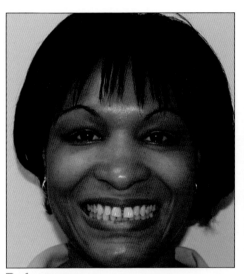

Before

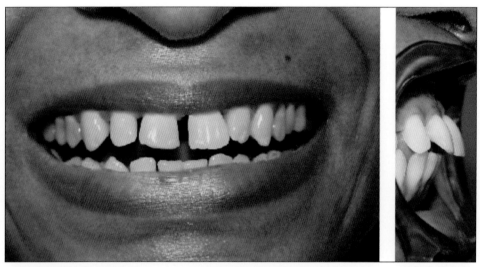

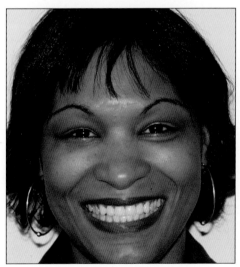

After

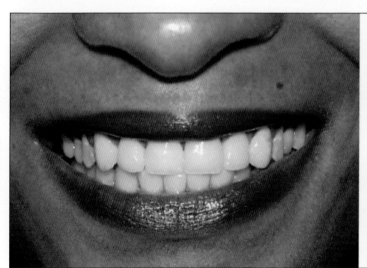

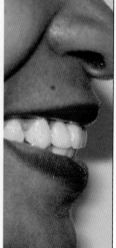

With the help of ten porcelain veneers and in-office bleaching, her smile was restored in two visits.

WORN INCISAL EDGES

Here we see that the edges of her maxillary four incisors are extremely worn and teeth are yellow.

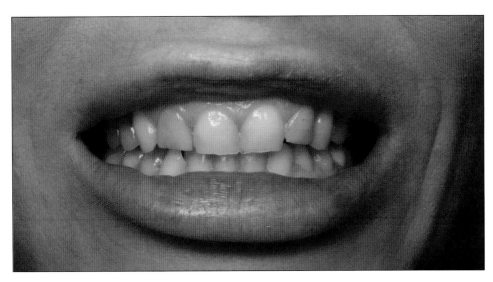

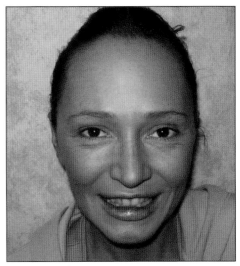

Before

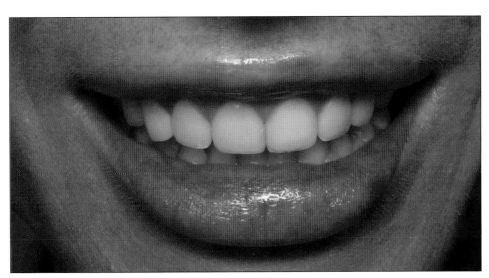

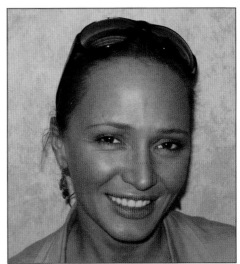

After

By placing eight porcelain veneers, she was able to restore her four incisors and broaden the look of her smile. What a difference!

CROOKED, CHIPPED AND GRAY TEETH

Here we have a combination of gray teeth, crooked teeth and chipped teeth.
He wanted an attractive smile.

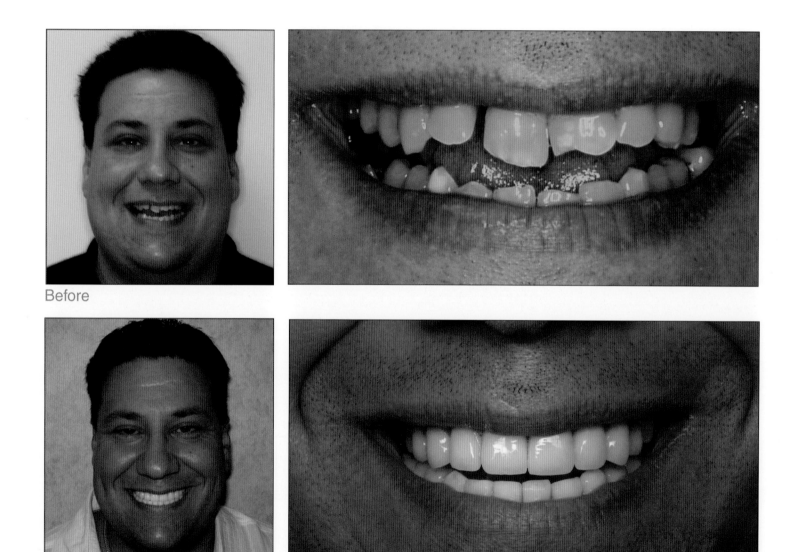

Before

After

With the help of 18 veneers in just two visits, he got just the smile he had always wanted.

NO ROOM FOR LATERAL INCISOR

Here we have a severely constricted arch with no room for her maxillary right lateral incisor. It was pushed in towards the tongue. This patient did not want to spend two years in orthodontic treatment.

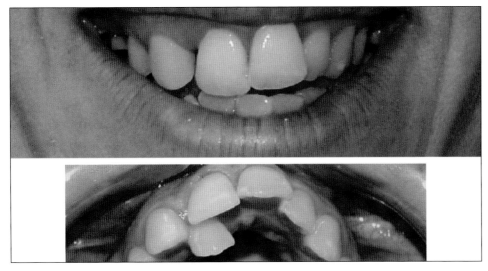
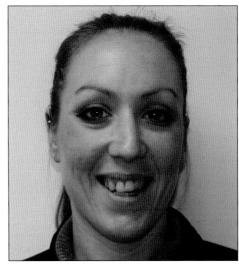

Before

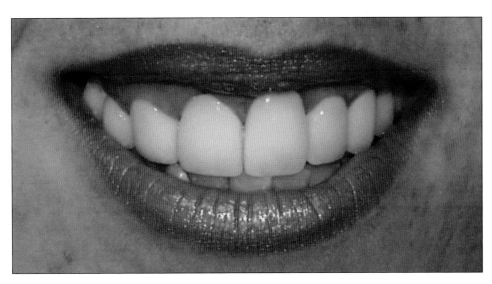
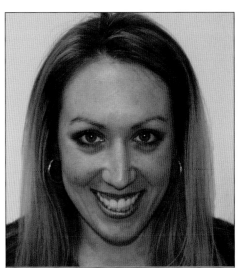

After

Once the lateral incisor was removed, her teeth were restored with eight porcelain veneers. Her right canine was shaped like a lateral incisor and her right first bicuspid was shaped like a canine.

PROGNATHIC MANDIBLE

Here we see a patient with a prognathic mandible (his lower teeth were forward and in front of upper teeth). Correction would have required extensive maxillofacial surgery and orthodontic treatment.

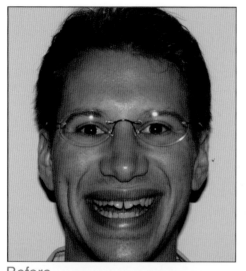
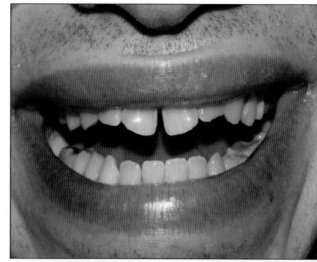
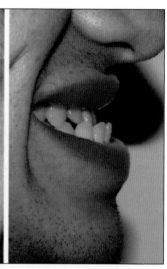

Before

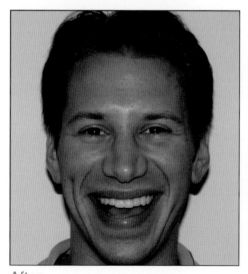
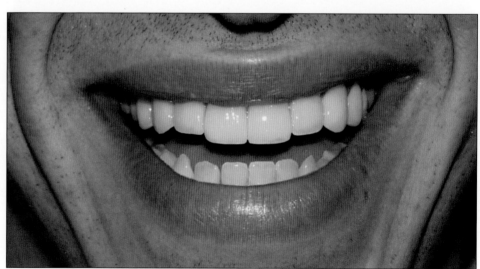

After

It's hard to believe that his cosmetic problem was solved with eight porcelain veneers in just two visits.

MISSING MANY TEETH

This patient was missing all her upper teeth and many of her lower teeth.
This prematurely aged her facial features, making her look older.
Notice how the lips cave in and wrinkle.

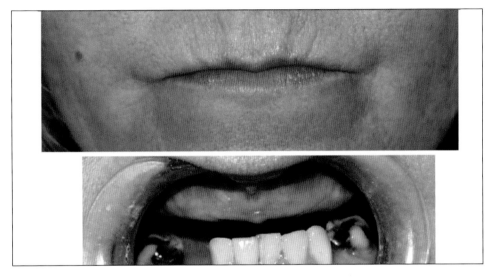
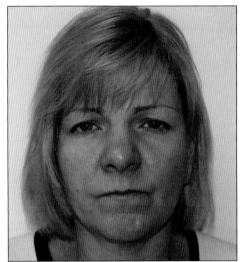

Before

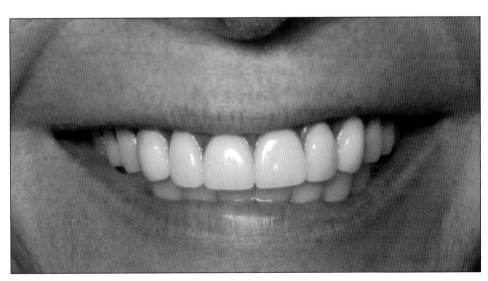
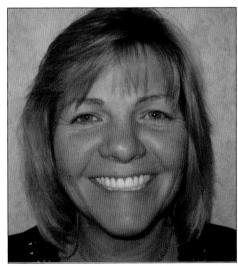

After

By placing dental implants, her mouth was able to be fully restored. Besides improving her ability to chew foods that she missed, her youthful facial features returned.

DECAYED AND CROOKED TEETH

Decayed and crooked teeth really detracted from this young woman's smile.

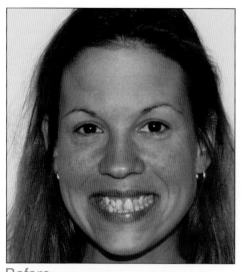

Before

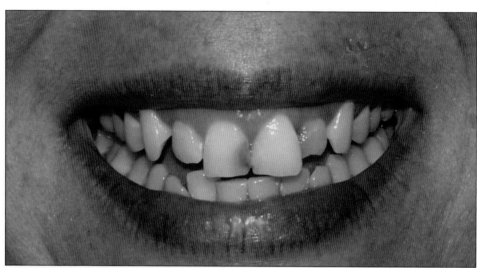

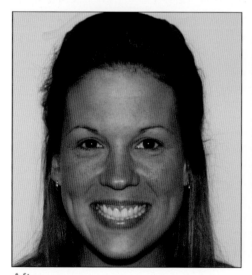

After

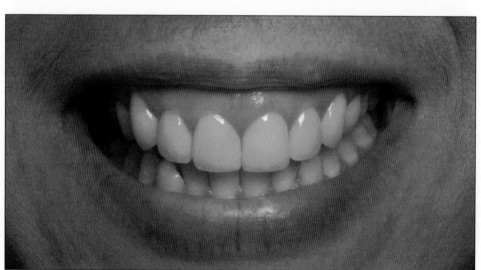

After removing all the tooth decay, eight porcelain veneers were placed, changing her smile forever in a mere two visits.

SPACED AND DRIFTING TEETH

This woman noticed her right central incisor moving forward over time while spaces were developing around the other anterior teeth.

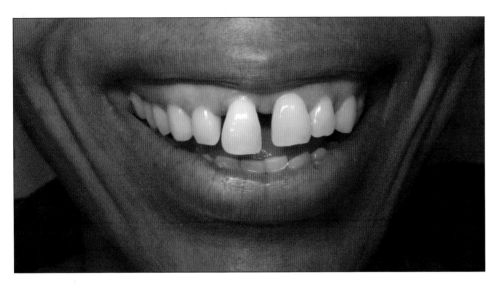
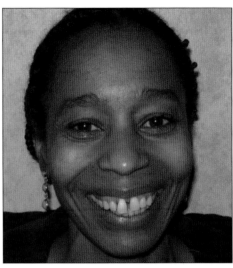

Before

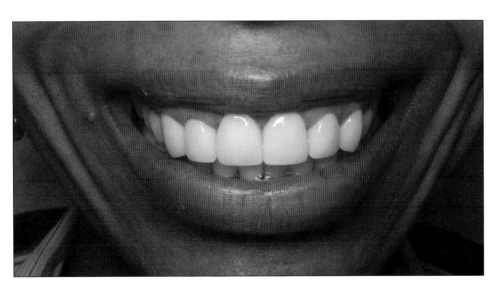
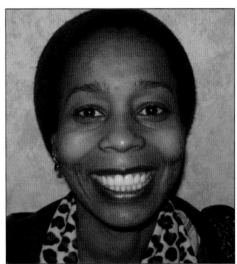

After

With six porcelain veneers, she was able to get her incisors back in line and eliminate those spaces that always bothered her.

SHORT TEETH

This young man always felt self conscious about his short maxillary teeth. He wanted to show more tooth structure when he smiled.

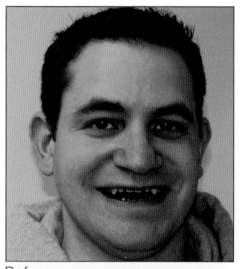

Before

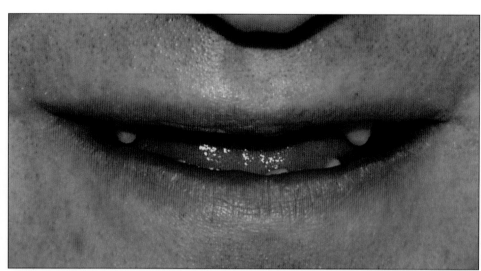

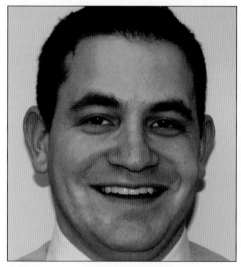

After

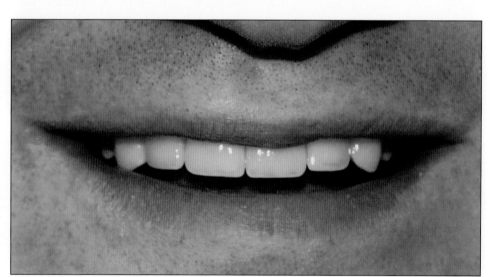

With just six porcelain veneers, he was able to attain that smile he had always imagined.

DARK ROOT CANAL TEETH

This woman's two front teeth received root canal treatment years earlier.
Over time they had become dark. She also wanted to get rid of her "pointy" canines
and rounded lateral incisors.

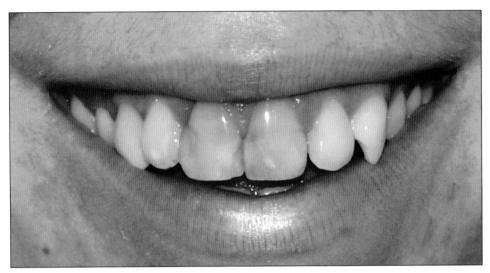

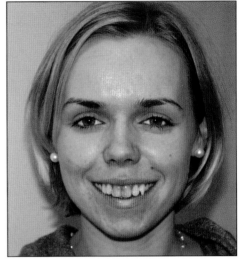

Before

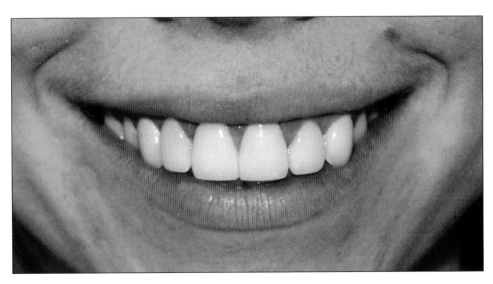

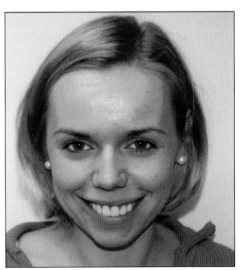

After

By making two all ceramic crowns for her central incisors and placing four porcelain
veneers on the lateral incisors and canines, her smile was restored.

DECAYED TEETH AND GUMMY SMILE

Here we see a gummy smile, decayed, crooked teeth and hypocalifications (white spots).

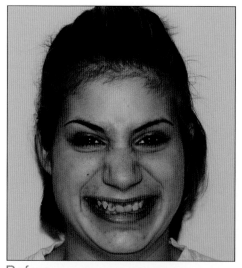

Before

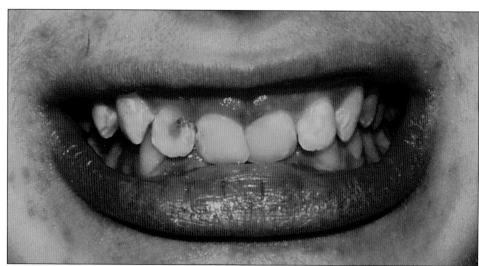

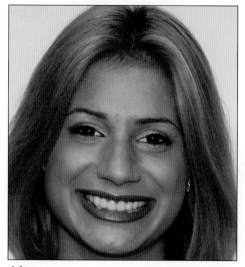

After

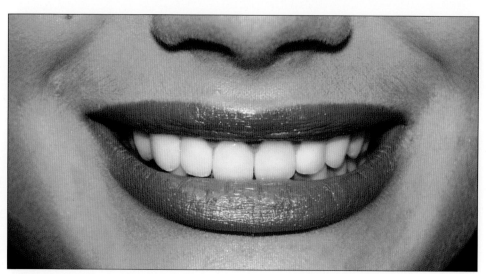

Crown lengthening surgery was performed over her four anterior teeth.
This was followed by eight porcelain veneers.

LARGE DIASTEMA

The large space between the two central incisors (called a diastema) always bothered this patient. She did not want to go through extensive orthodontic treatment.

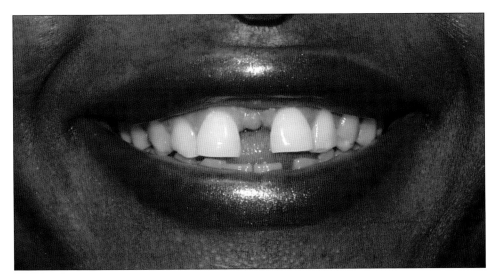
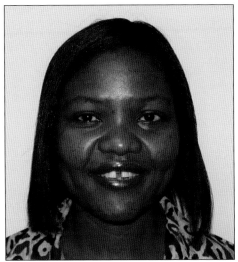

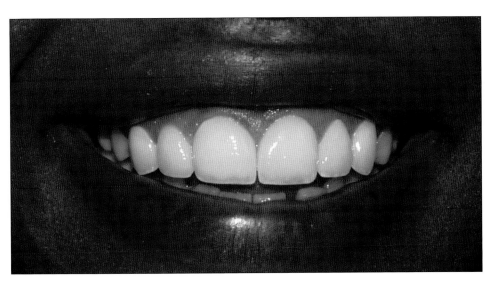
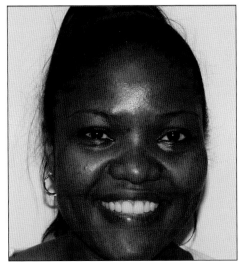

By placing just six porcelain veneers, her diastema was closed and a magnificent smile was created.

MISSING LATERAL INCISOR

Unfortunately, this young man lost his maxillary lateral incisor.

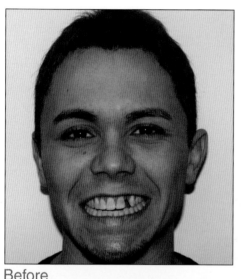

Before

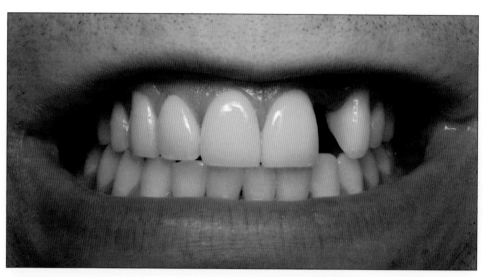

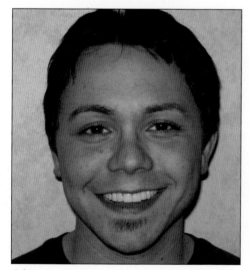

After

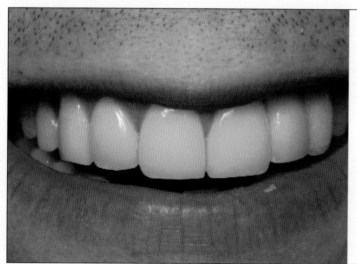

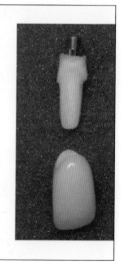

An implant was placed where the lateral incisor was lost. After the implant healed, a ceramic abutment was screwed into the implant. Finally, an all porcelain crown was placed on top of the abutment.

TRAUMATIC INJURY TO FRONT TEETH

A traumatic injury to the maxillary anterior incisors left the edges chipped, disfiguring this woman's otherwise perfect smile.

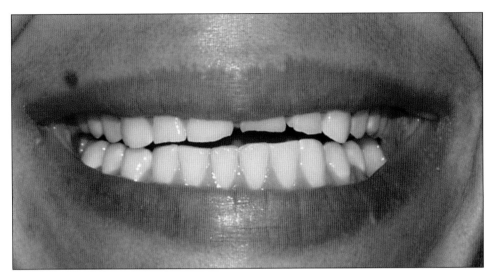

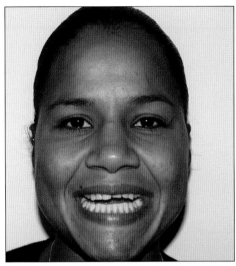

Before

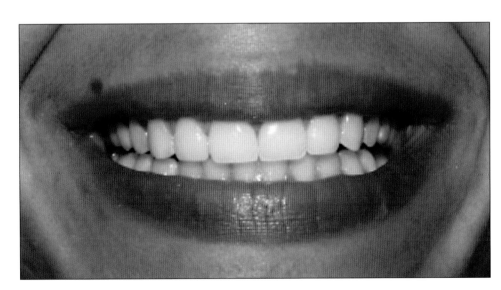

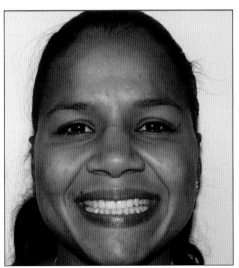

After

With six beautiful porcelain veneers, her magnificent smile was restored in just one week.

DISCOLORED TEETH MAKE YOU LOOK OLDER

This woman wanted to revitalize her face. Her first step was to remove old and discolored bonded restorations.

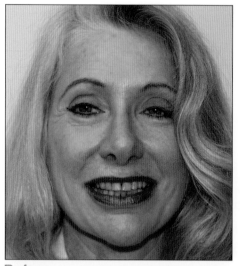
Before

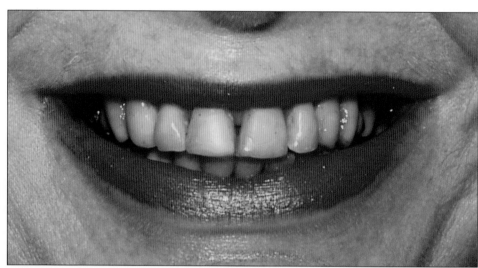

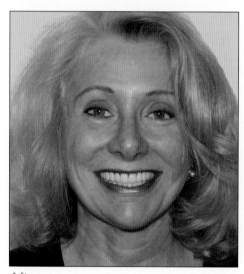
After

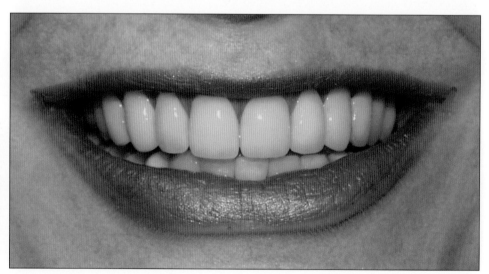

By placing 18 porcelain veneers and three porcelain crowns, a more youthful smile returned, making her look 10 years younger.

WORN INCISAL EDGES

Severe teeth grinding destroyed this patient's smile and collapsed his bite.

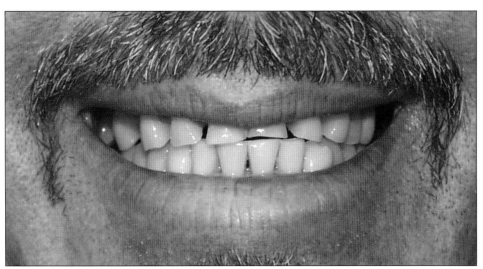
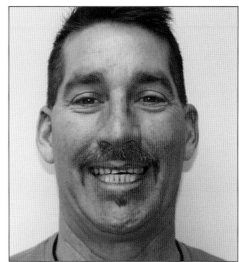

Before

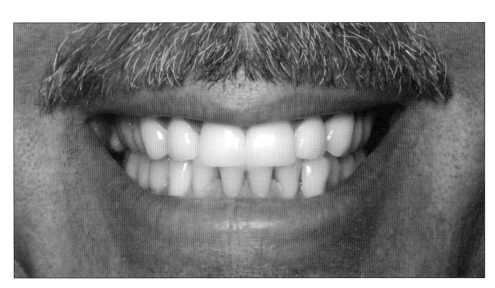
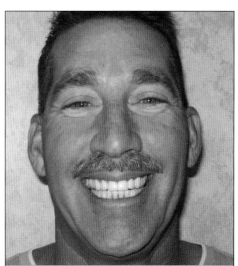

After

By restoring his upper teeth with twelve porcelain-fused-to-metal crowns, his bite was corrected and smile regained.

NARROW ARCH WITH OLD BONDED TEETH

This patient wanted more teeth to show when she smiled.

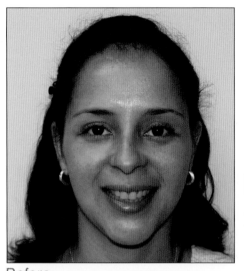

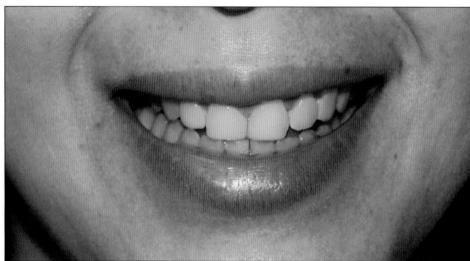

Before

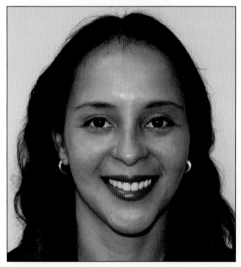

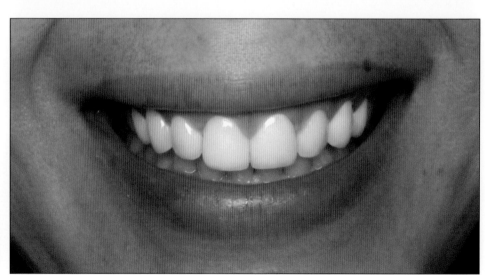

After

The old bonding material was removed from her teeth. The smile was made wider by using eight porcelain veneers.

OLD DENTAL RESTORATIONS

This young woman had old porcelain-fused-to-metal bridges and old unsightly bonded restorations. She wanted a more youthful and energetic smile.

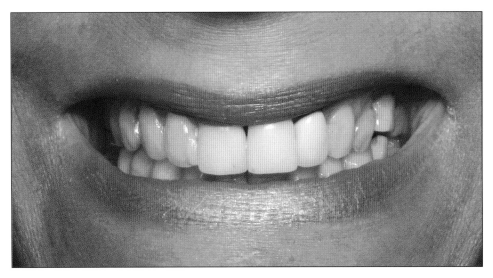
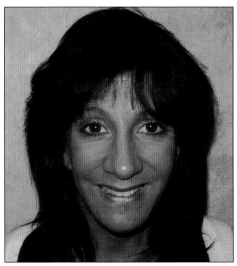

Before

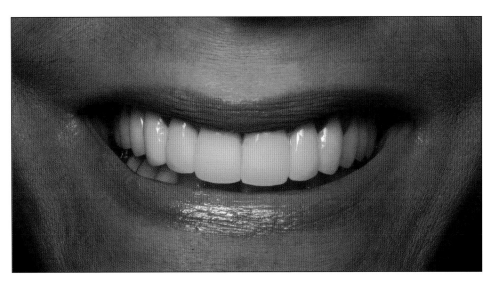
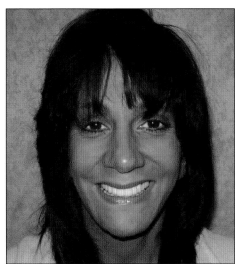

After

She was able to get exactly what she wanted with all porcelain bridges complimented by all porcelain crowns.

ADVANCED DENTAL BREAKDOWN

This young woman suffered from advanced decay resulting in loss of all her upper teeth.
Her lower teeth were decayed to the gum line.

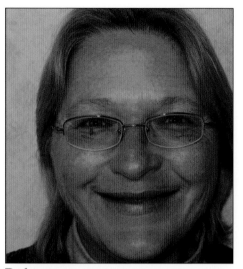

Before

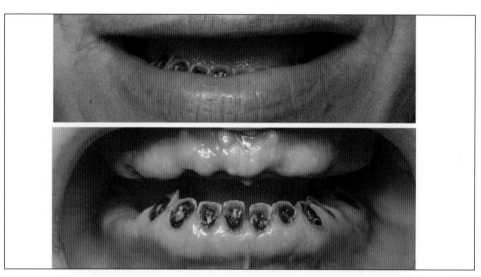

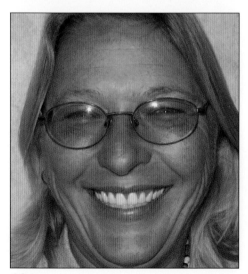

After

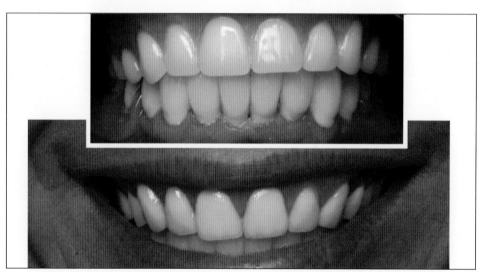

By placing dental implants in her upper jaw, the maxillary teeth were easily restored.
Her lower teeth were restored with porcelain-fused-to-metal crowns and a partial denture.

UNBALANCED LOOKING MAXILLARY TEETH

Sometimes not all anterior teeth require veneers. Here we have a situation with small and slightly intruded lateral incisors and pointy canine teeth.

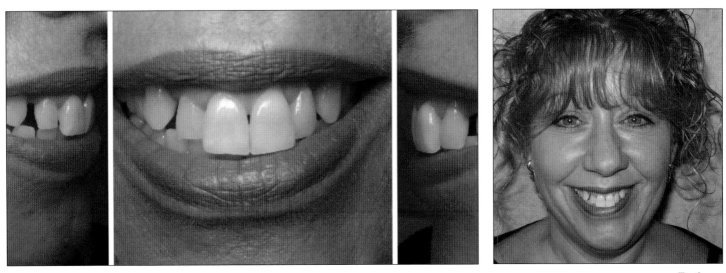

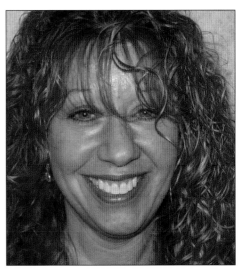

Before

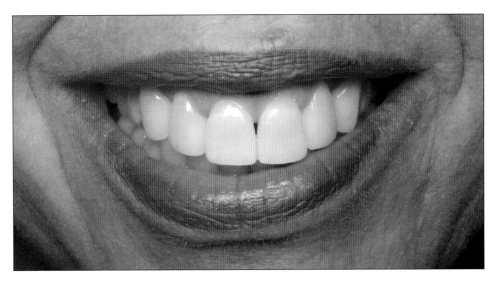

After

Her concerns were satisfied by placing four porcelain veneers
on the lateral incisors and canines.

DARK, CROOKED AND WORN TEETH

Here we have a combination of smile detractors. This patient has worn and yellow teeth, crooked teeth and unmatched lower posterior crowns. Dark tunnels on each side of the smile make his maxillary arch seem narrow.

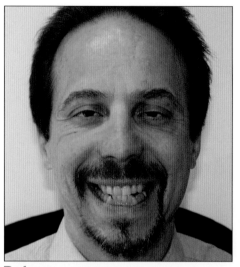
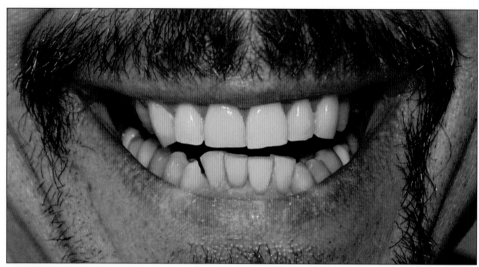

Before

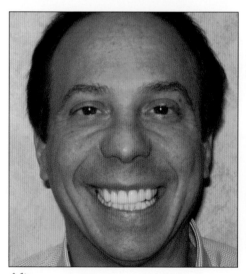
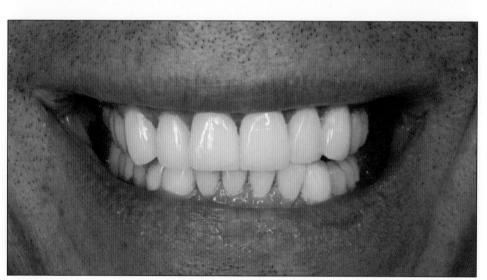

After

It's amazing how so many problems can be corrected with ten porcelain veneers and four porcelain crowns in just two visits.

MISSING LATERAL INCISORS & RETAINED BABY TEETH

This young girl had congenitally missing lateral incisors. Her canines moved into their position. In the back of her mouth, she was missing bicuspids and retained her primary teeth, thereby giving her an immature smile.

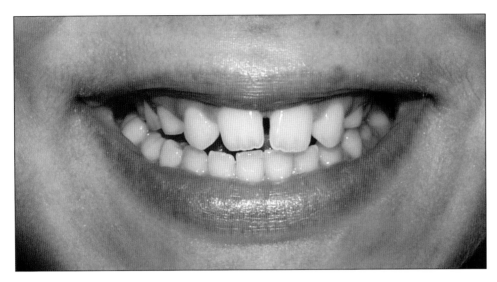 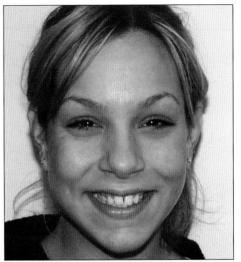

Before

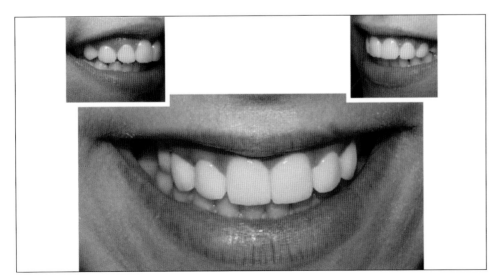 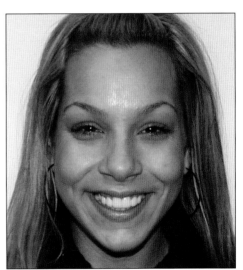

After

After she had her primary (baby) teeth removed, her smile was restored with two porcelain veneers and two all porcelain bridges.

CROOKED TEETH

This man was leaving for overseas and did not have the time to straighten his teeth with traditional orthodontic treatment.

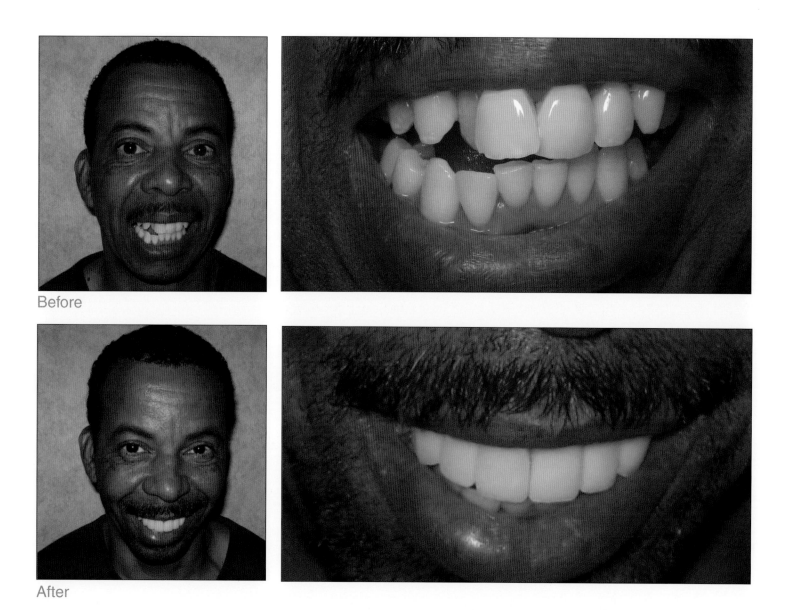

Before

After

The solution was placing six porcelain veneers, in just two visits.

TETRACYCLINE STAINED TEETH

This mouth shows classic tetracycline stained teeth. There is also slight overlapping of her central incisors and a crooked right lateral incisor.

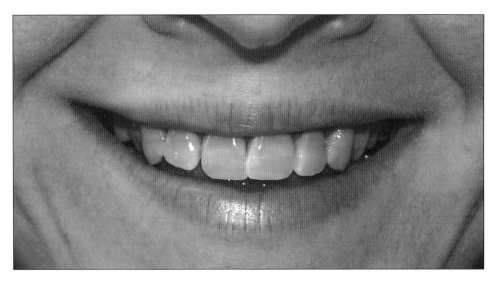

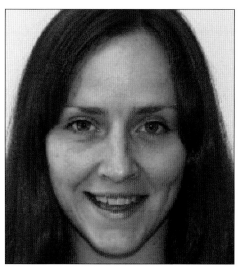

Before

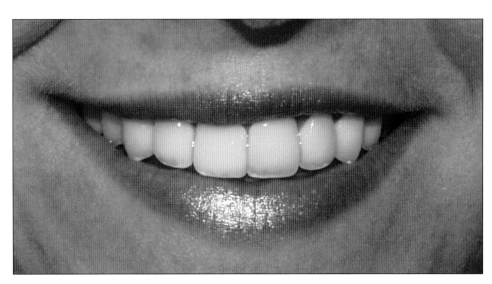

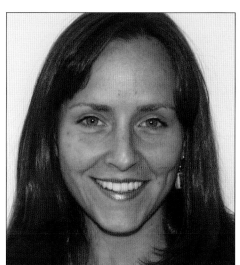

After

The entire problem was solved quickly with ten porcelain veneers.

SHORT AND WORN MAXILLARY TEETH

This woman did not like to smile because her maxillary teeth were short with worn edges.

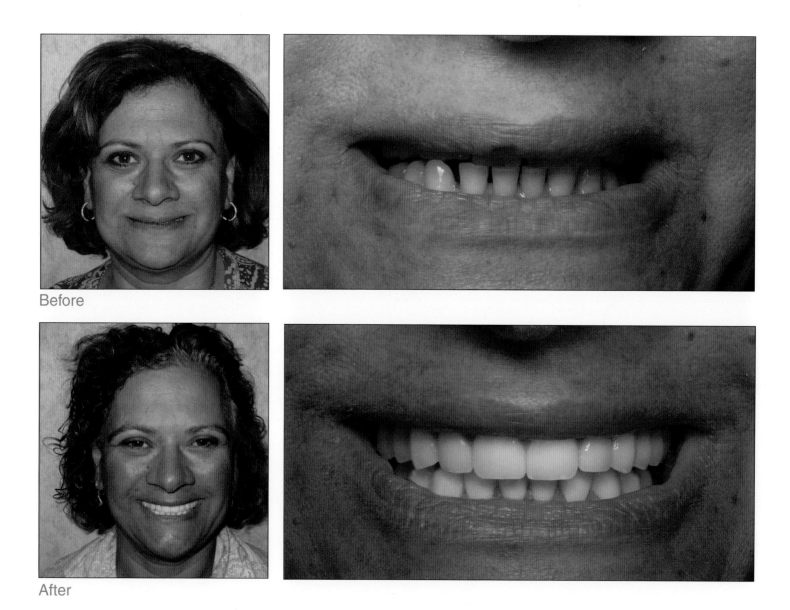

Before

After

By placing a combination of porcelain crowns and porcelain veneers, her teeth were lengthened and her smile was greatly improved.

PROGNATHIC MANDIBLE

A severely prognathic lower jaw hides his upper short teeth.
This patient needed a quick solution to a complex cosmetic problem.

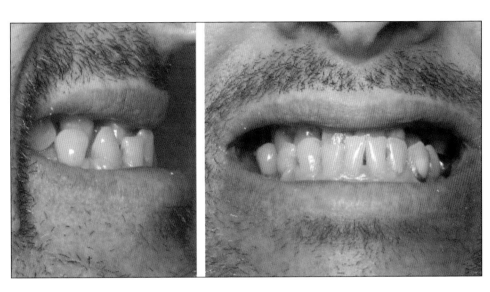 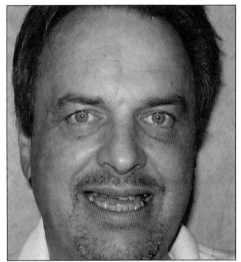

Before

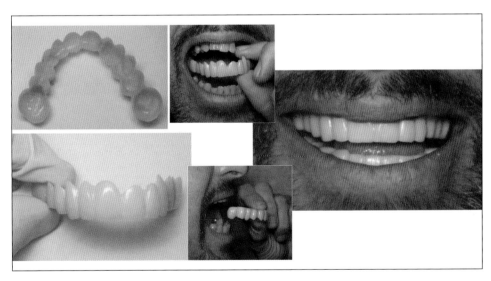 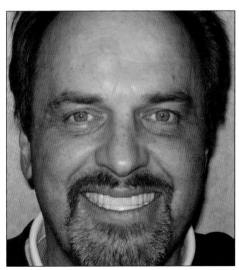

After

By using a two visit procedure called a "snap on smile", this gentleman was able to have a new smile in two weeks. When his schedule permits, he will replace this temporary snap on smile with permanent porcelain crowns.

PROGNATHIC MANDIBLE

A severely prognathic lower jaw hides his upper short teeth.
This patient needed a quick solution to a complex cosmetic problem.

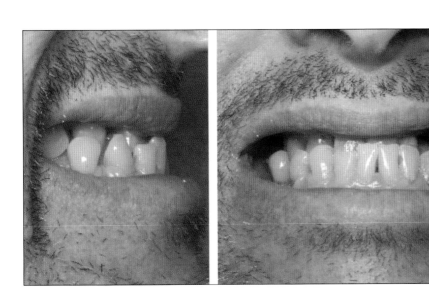

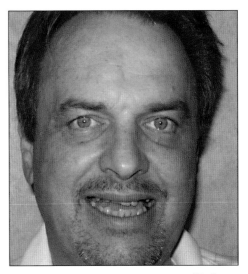
Before

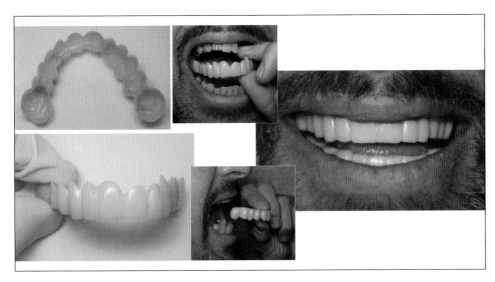

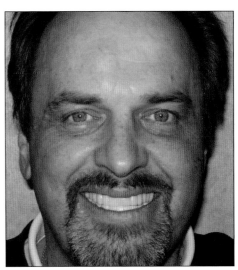
After

By using a two visit procedure called a "snap on smile", this gentleman was able to have a new smile in two weeks. When his schedule permits, he will replace this temporary snap on smile with permanent porcelain crowns.

AN UNSIGHTLY SMILE

A combination of stained, twisted and worn teeth has detracted from this patient's smile.

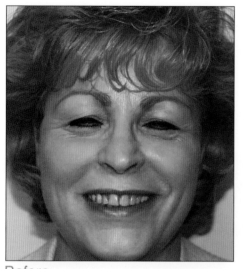

Before

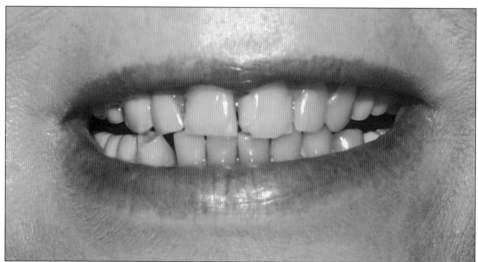

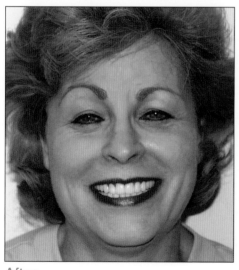

After

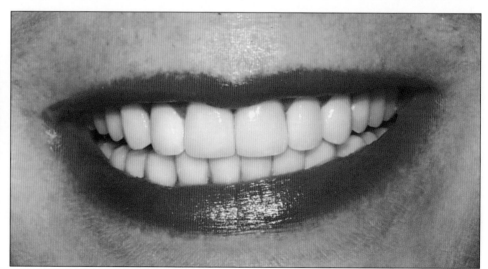

By repairing and replacing the teeth with porcelain veneers and bridges,
a younger smile returned.

MISSING FRONT TEETH

Missing front teeth always detracts from a smile.

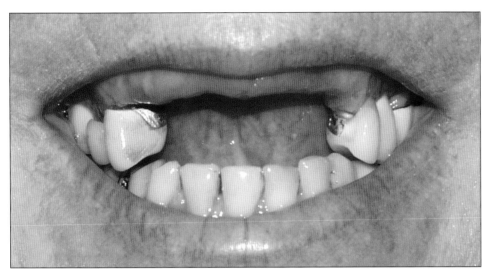

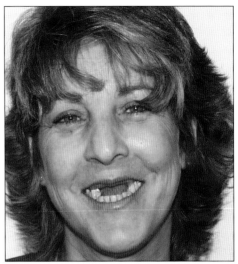

Before

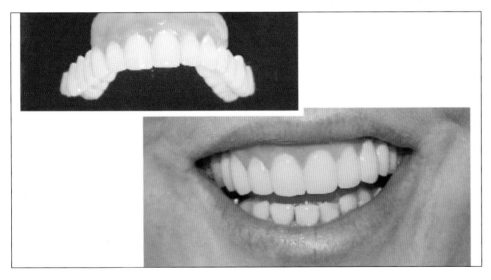

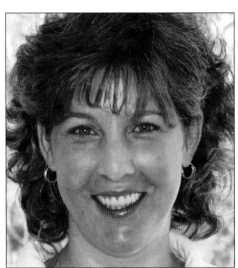

After

The problem was solved with a full arch, "round house," porcelain-fused-to-gold bridge.
Pink porcelain was also utilized to simulate the missing gum tissue.
She now has a beautiful smile!

CROOKED UPPER RIGHT TEETH

This young man always disliked his canine "fang". The tooth in front and back of it were too far into his mouth. He was told that he needed two years of orthodontic treatment.

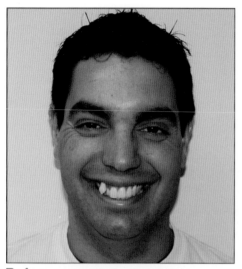

Before

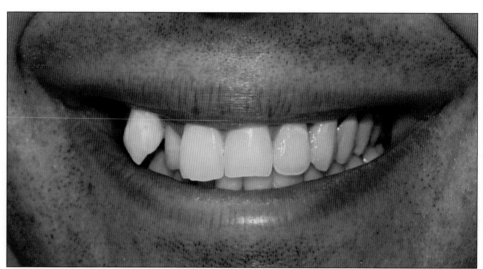

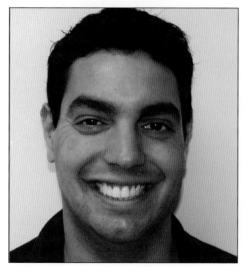

After

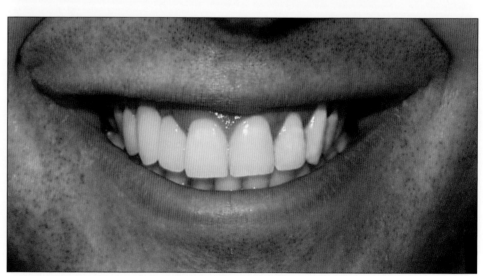

Instead he opted for a root canal on the canine followed by three porcelain veneers.
Treatment time… three visits!

ADVANCED PERIODONTAL DISEASE

Periodontal disease caused this patient to lose his four front incisors
and much of his gum tissue.

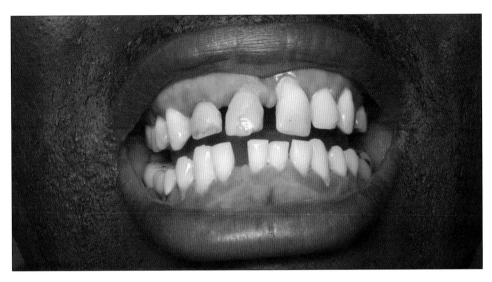
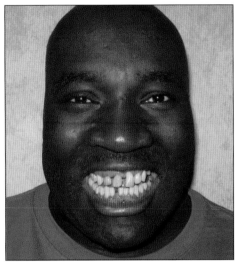

Before

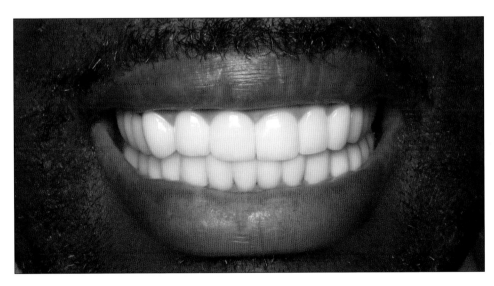
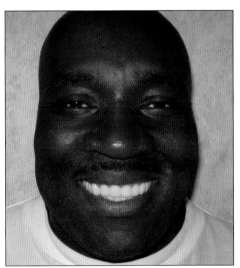

After

After periodontal treatment, his teeth were replaced with porcelain-fused-to-metal crowns
and his gums were replaced with pink porcelain.

DECAY AND GUMMY SMILE

This young woman had advanced decay and a very gummy smile.

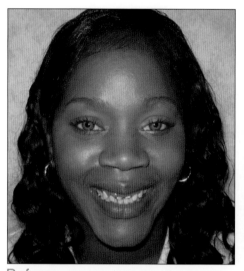

Before

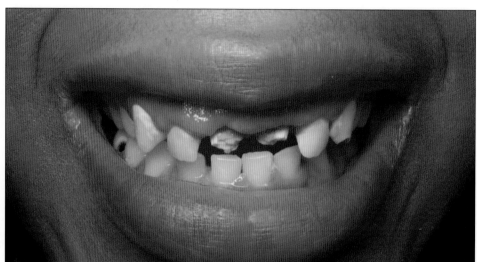

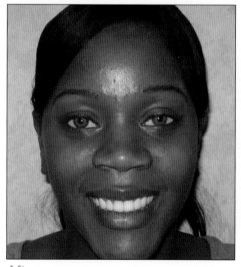

After

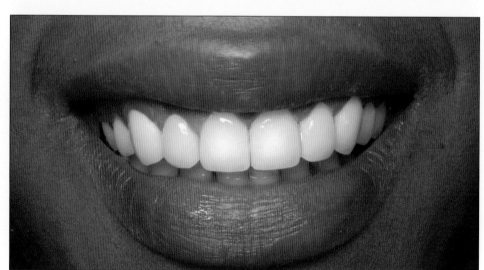

A gingivectomy was performed to reduce extra gum tissue. Two all porcelain crowns were placed on her central incisors and eight porcelain veneers were placed on the other maxillary teeth. Now she has that smile she always wanted.

ADVANCED DENTAL DISEASE

This young woman had advanced decay and teeth broken down to the gum line.
She just wanted her smile back.

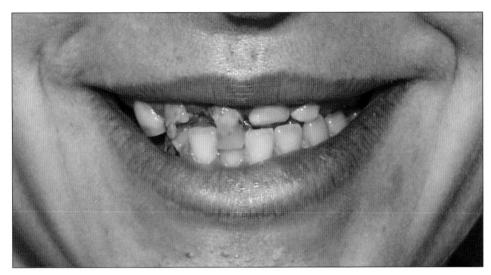
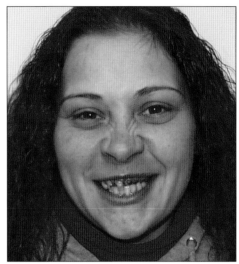

Before

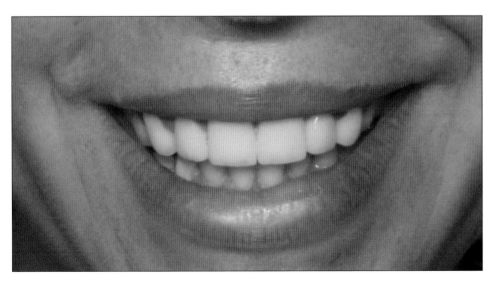
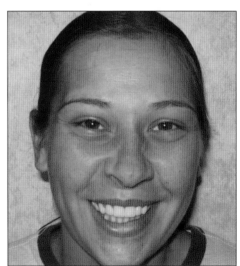

After

Her smile ultimately returned after minor gum treatment, bonded fillings
and twelve porcelain-fused-to-metal crowns.

WORN TEETH FROM YEARS OF GRINDING

This young man suffered from night grinding which ultimately wore his teeth down through the enamel layer, resulting in a collapsed bite.

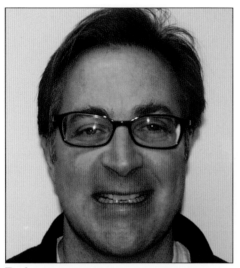

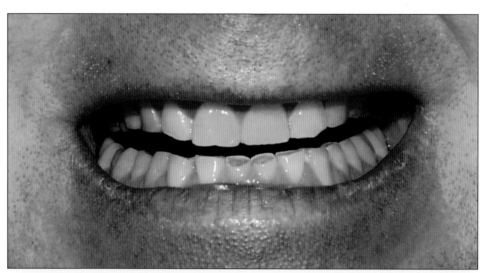

Before

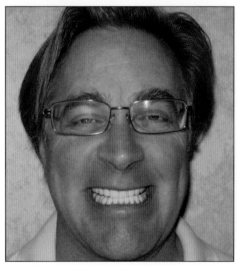

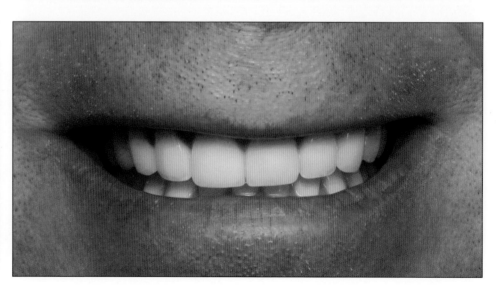

After

By raising his bite with porcelain onlays and porcelain crowns,
his natural smile was re-established.

MISSING MAXILLARY POSTERIOR TEETH

Here is an example of broken down anterior teeth with missing posterior maxillary teeth.

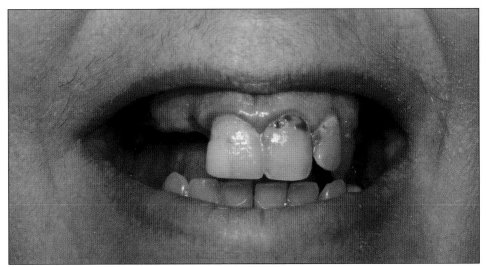
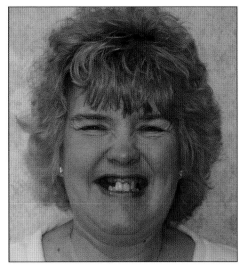

Before

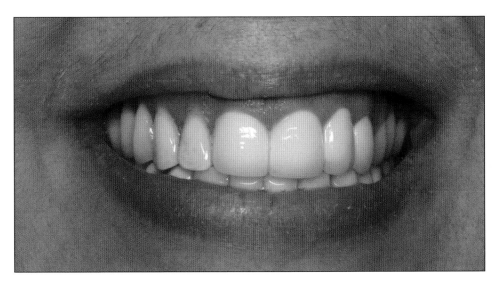
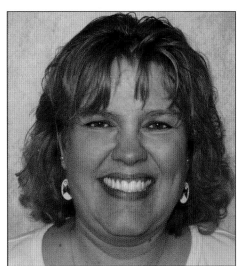

After

By restoring the anterior teeth with porcelain-fused-to-gold crowns that contained invisible attachments, posterior teeth could be replaced with a removable appliance that could not be detected.

WORN TEETH AND GUMMY SMILE

This young woman grinds her teeth at night which has resulted in worn incisal edges.

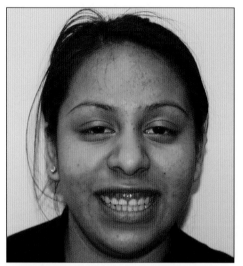

Before

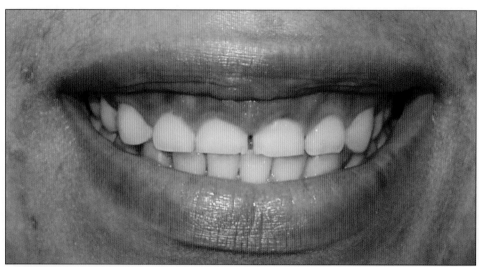

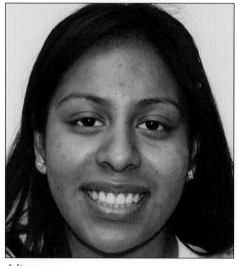

After

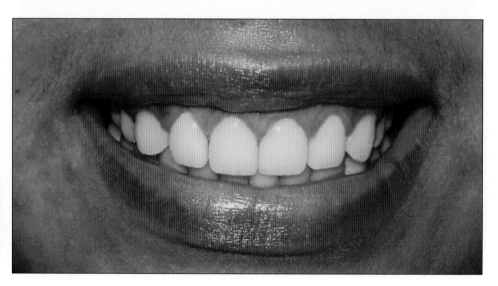

A gum lift surgery was performed to reduce extra gum tissue. Six porcelain veneers were then placed on her six maxillary incisors to re-establish her natural smile.

UNILATERAL ANTERIOR OPEN BITE

When this patient smiles, his front left lateral incisor is too short which creates a dark space between his upper and lower arches.

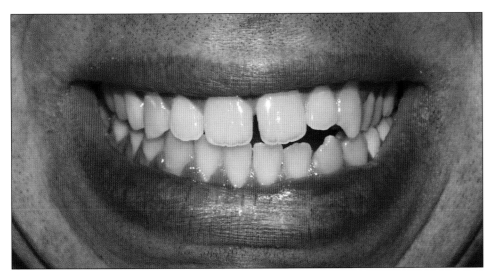
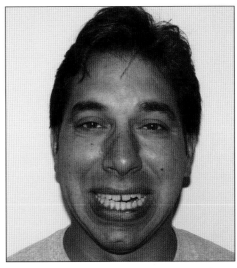

Before

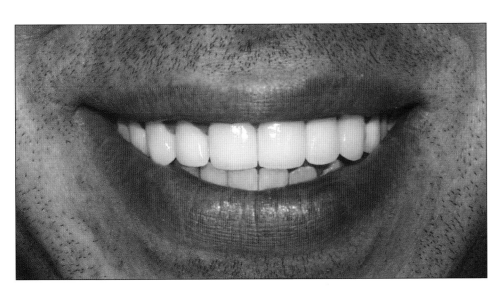
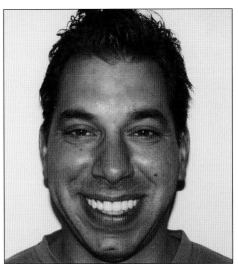

After

With porcelain veneers, the problem was easily corrected in two visits.

MISSING LATERAL INCISORS

This young woman had her missing lateral incisors replaced with Maryland bridges.
Notice how the opaque looking pontics do not match the natural teeth.

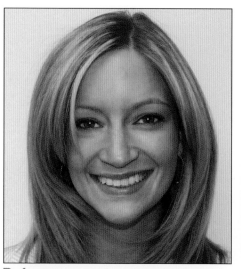

Before

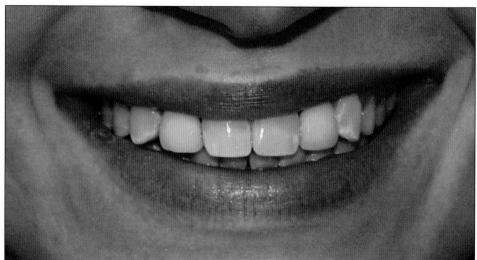

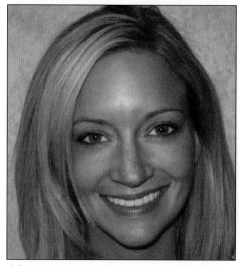

After

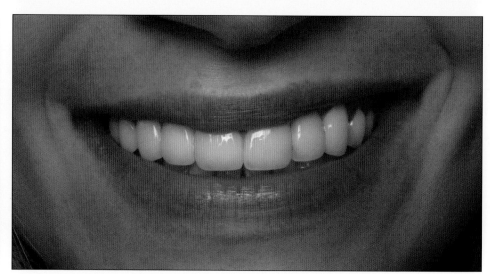

Two all porcelain bridges were placed along with four additional porcelain veneers.
Her smile was improved in three visits.

CROOKED TEETH AND SPACES

Here we have twisted teeth, worn incisal edges and spaces between her teeth.

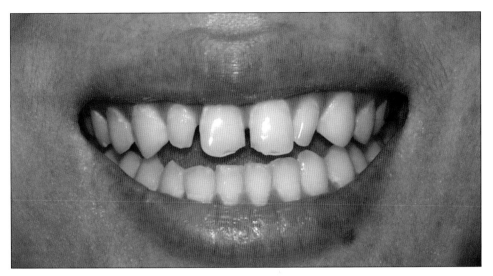

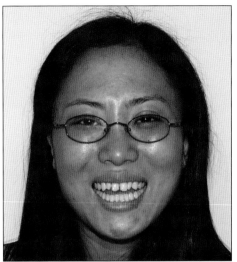

Before

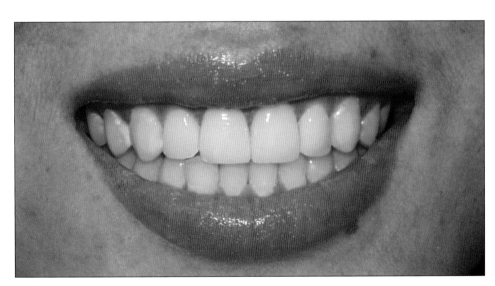

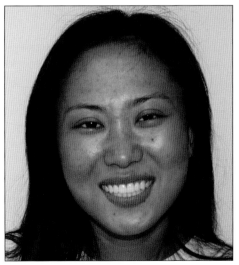

After

By placing just four porcelain veneers, her smile was dramatically improved in one week.

WORN EDGES MAKE SMILES LOOK OLDER

Not only do worn edges on teeth look unsightly, they also make a person look older.

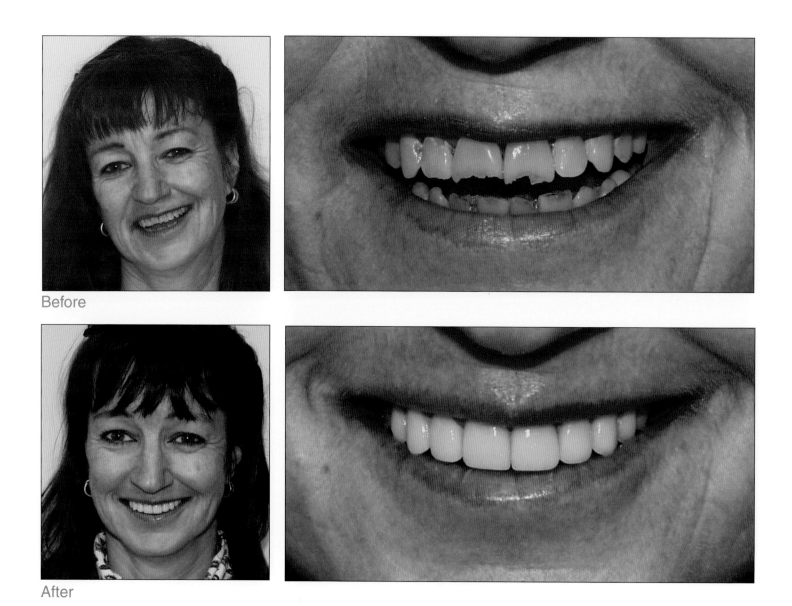

Before

After

By placing eight porcelain veneers, an attractive and much younger
looking smile was attained.

ADVANCED MALOCCLUSION

Her lateral incisors are in severe cross bite and canines are sticking out.
This patient did not want to go through major orthodontic treatment.

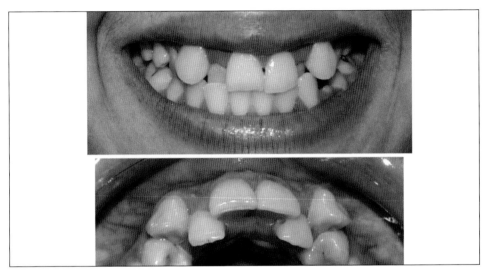
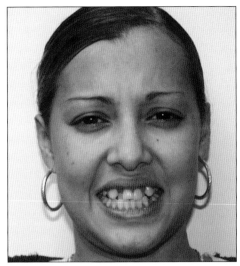

Before

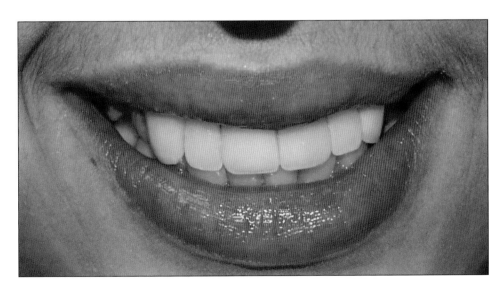
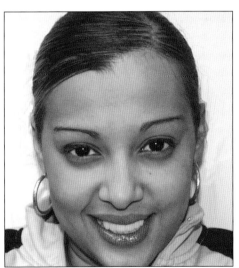

After

She had root canal treatment on her lateral incisors so that they could be
repositioned. This was followed by ceramic posts and six porcelain veneers.
Entire treatment time was three visits!

UNDERDEVELOPED MAXILLARY TEETH

Here is a case where the maxillary teeth did not fully erupt and the maxillary bone was underdeveloped, resulting in an underbite.

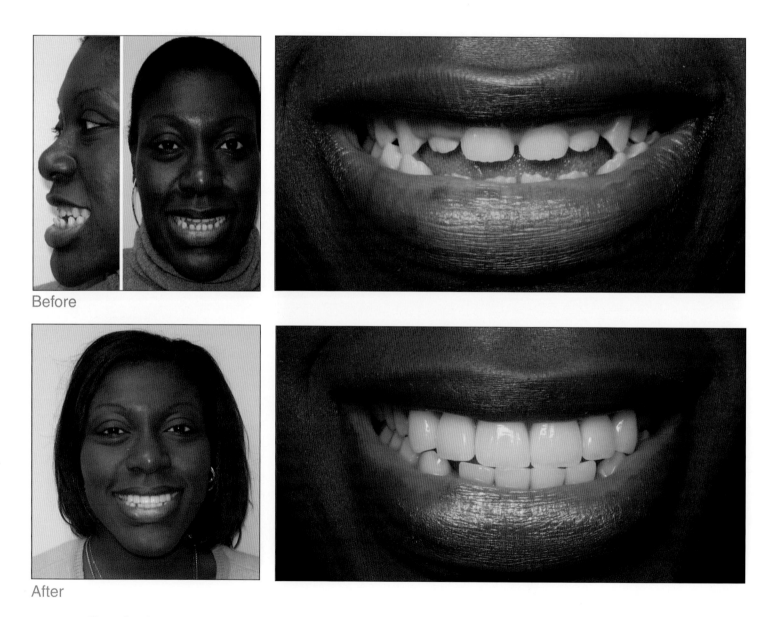

Before

After

By placing ten veneers, her underbite was restored and her profile improved.

OLD BRIDGE NEEDS REPLACING

The gums are inflamed around her failing upper right bridge.
The rest of the smile needs to be brightened.

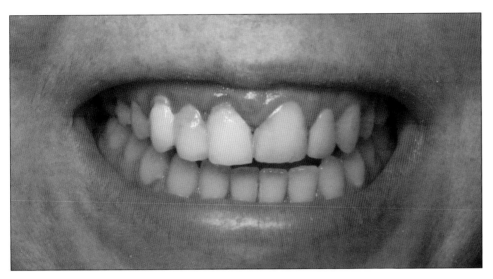

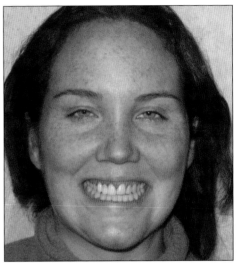

Before

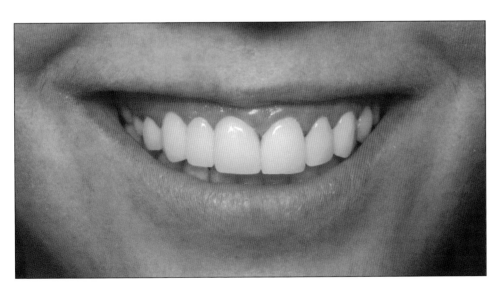

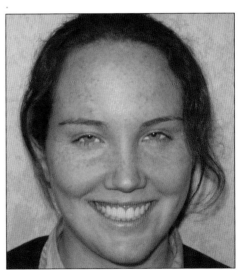

After

Her inflamed gums received periodontal treatment. An all porcelain three unit bridge was placed with five porcelain veneers. What a greatly improved smile.

ADVANCED TOOTH BREAKDOWN

Advanced decay and wear totally destroyed the look of this young woman's smile.

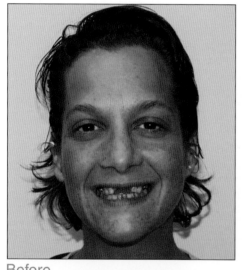

Before

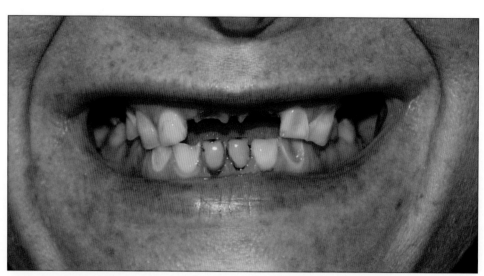

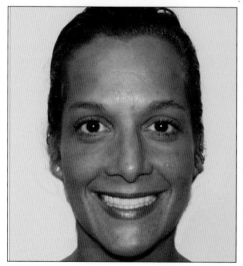

After

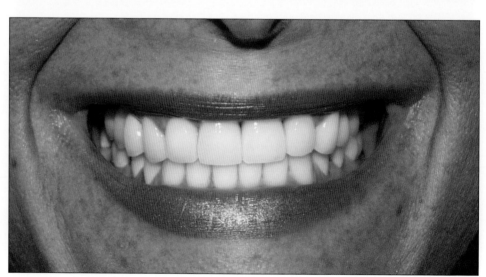

Using porcelain crowns and porcelain veneers,
her smile and beauty were restored in just a couple of visits.

A YOUNGER LOOKING SMILE

Years of wear and staining made this patient's smile and face look older.

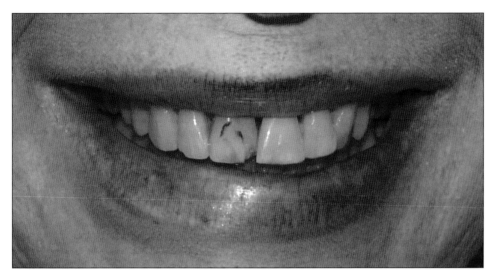

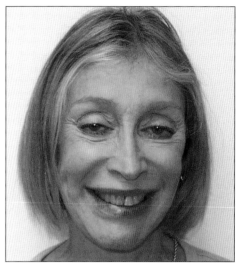

Before

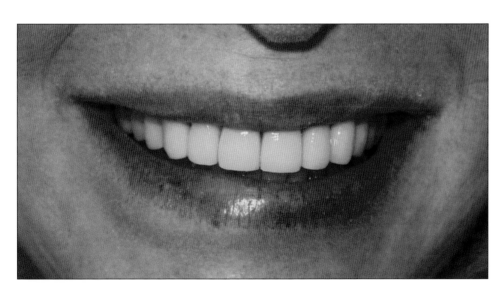

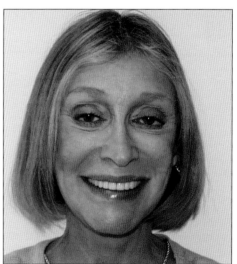

After

It took just twelve porcelain veneers and two visits to get that youthful smile back.

OVERLAPPING AND CROOKED TEETH

Here is another case where the patient did not want to go through long orthodontic treatment. He wanted a quicker alternative.

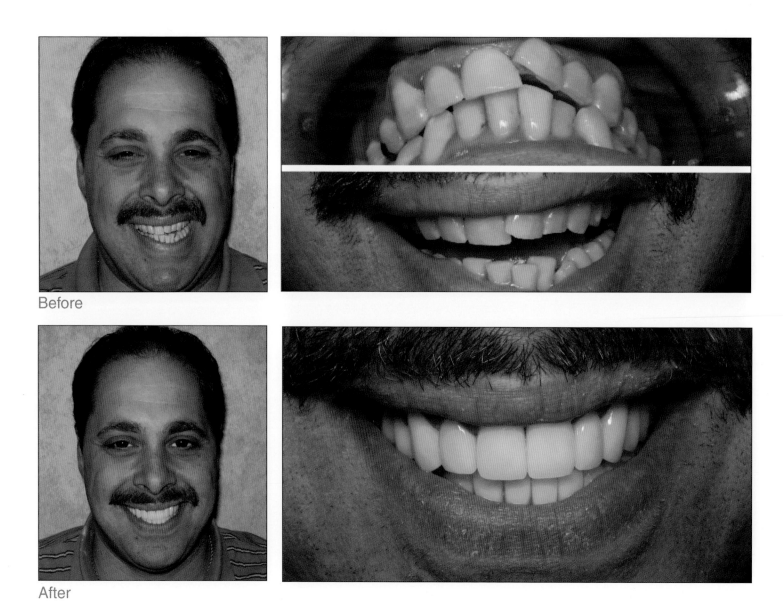

Before

After

The solution to his request was to make his teeth look straight by placing eighteen porcelain veneers in two visits.

MISSING PERMANENT TEETH

Several permanent teeth never erupted, leaving a combination of baby teeth and adult teeth in this young man's mouth. As he grew older, spaces appeared.

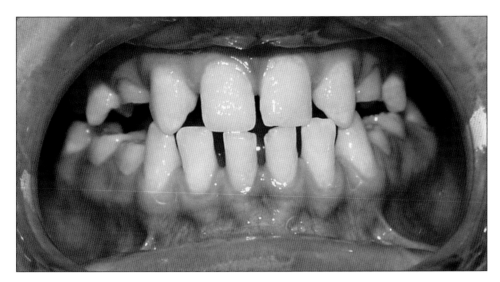
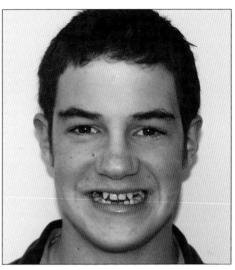

Before

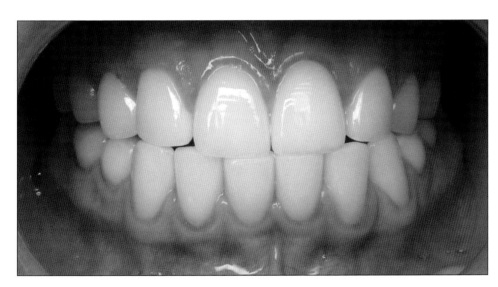
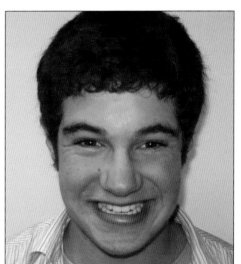

After

By using both porcelain veneers and porcelain crowns,
an attractive adult-looking smile was created.

MISMATCHED COLORS IN TEETH

Over the years, individual teeth can become different colors. This problem is caused by stains and by various dental treatments that were performed over time.

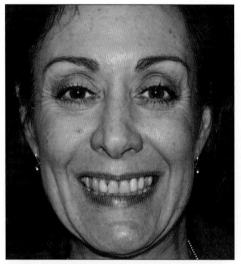
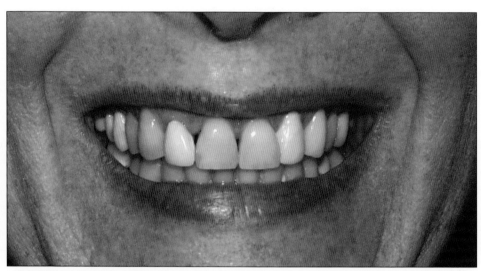

Before

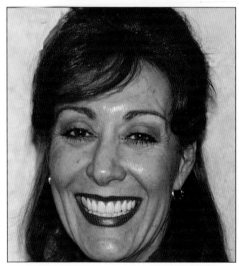
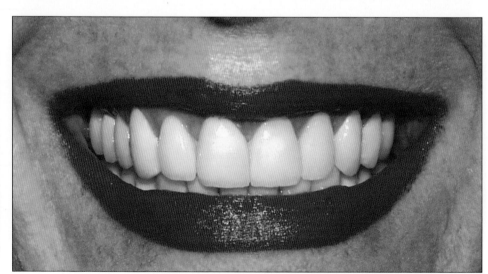

After

A more harmonious looking smile was established with porcelain veneers and porcelain crowns.

MISSING MAXILLARY CENTRAL & LATERAL INCISOR

This young man wanted his maxillary right central and
lateral incisors replaced and a brighter smile.

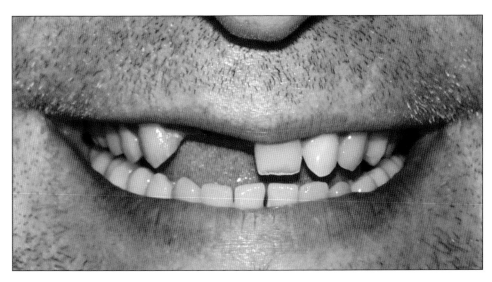

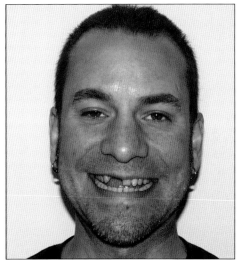

Before

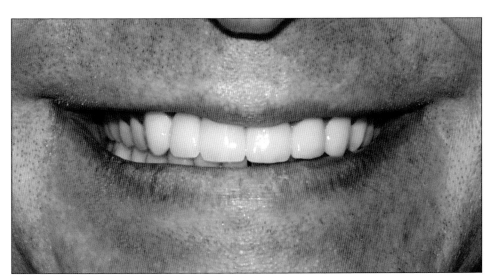

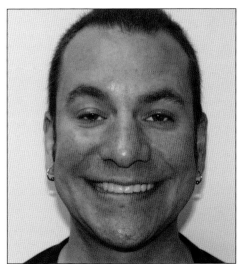

After

This was accomplished with a porcelain-fused-to-metal fixed bridge
and bleaching of his remaining teeth.

WHITE SPOTS (HYPOCALCIFICATIONS)

This patient had congenital white spots (hypocalcifications)
which were intensified after bleaching his teeth. He also wanted to correct the pointy
canines and lateral incisors.

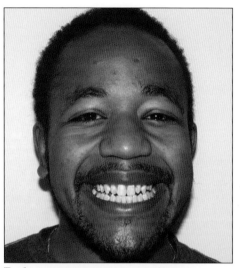

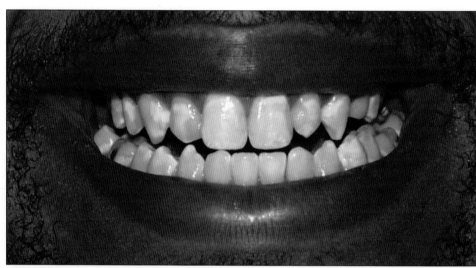

Before

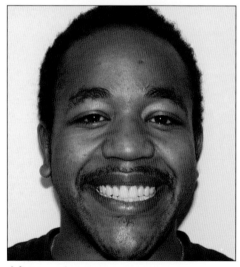

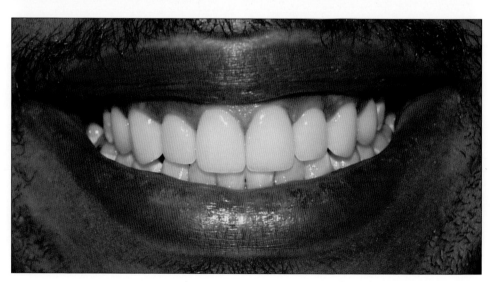

After

The problems were solved with eight porcelain veneers performed in two visits.
Now he loves his smile.

OLD BONDED TEETH

Over time, teeth that were once restored with bonding have now turned yellow
and show wear at the edges.

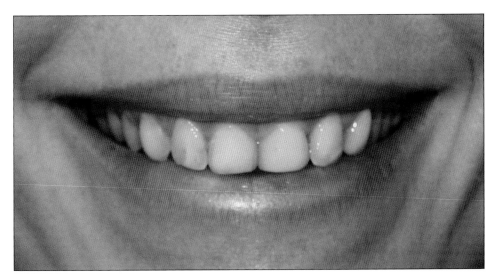

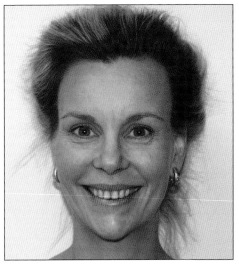

Before

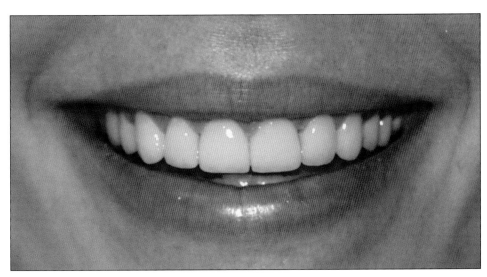

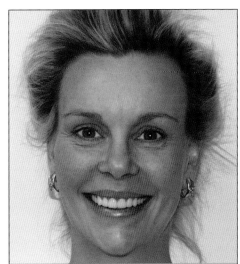

After

By replacing the old bonded restorations with ten porcelain veneers,
her beautiful smile was restored.

99

TOOTH ABRASION AND DECAY

This patient's teeth were severely worn from brushing too hard with a very abrasive tooth-paste. Once the protective outer enamel was perforated, decay followed. Her incisal edges were worn from grinding at night.

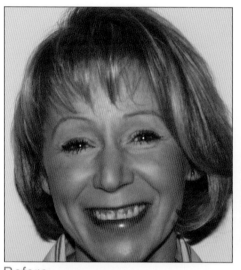

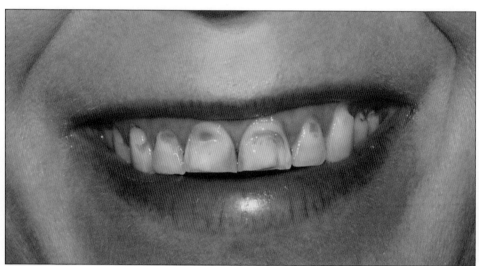

Before

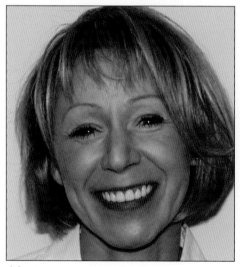

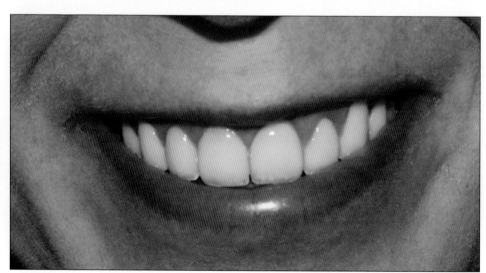

After

This unattractive smile was transformed into a beautiful smile by applying eight porcelain veneers in only three visits.

TETRACYCLINE STAINED TEETH

This young woman had her teeth stained by taking the antibiotic tetracycline as a child.

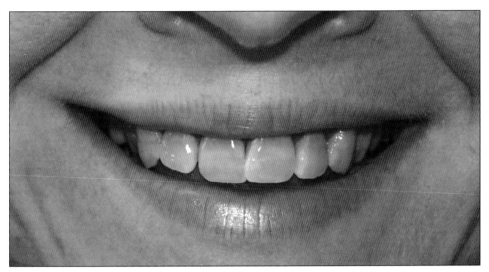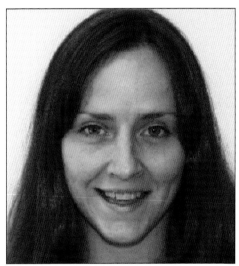

Before

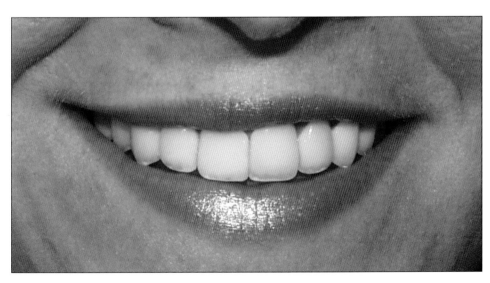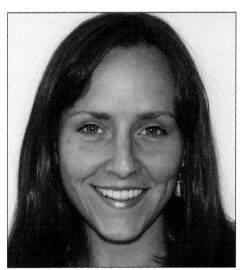

After

Although difficult to correct, ten porcelain veneers with a special built in opaque layer were able to block out the dark tooth color underneath.

GUMMY SMILE

Here we see a very gummy smile and teeth that are too small for her mouth and face.

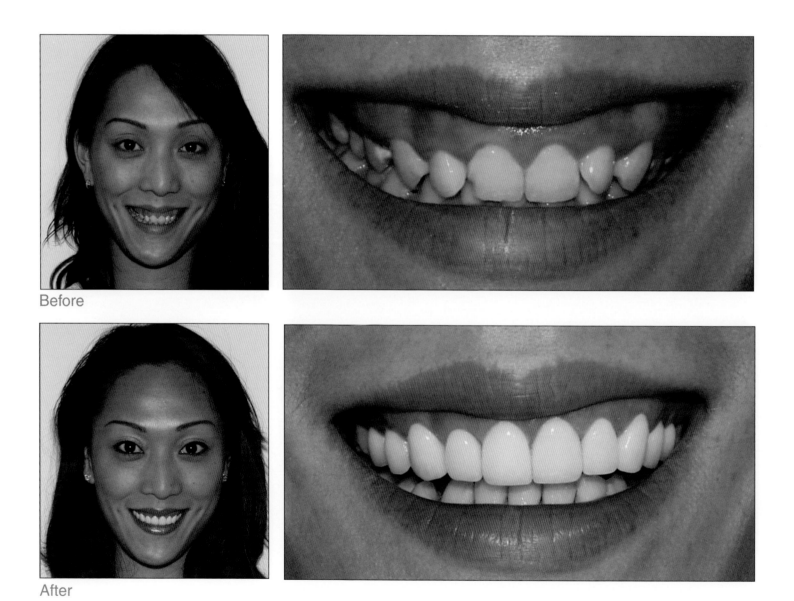

Before

After

This young lady was able to attain a radiant smile through a combination of gum lift surgery and porcelain veneers in four visits

TRAUMATIC INJURY

A traumatic injury to this young man's maxillary left central and lateral incisors ruined his smile.

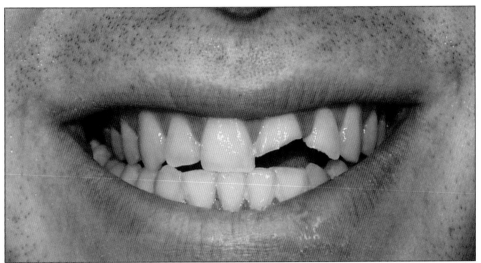

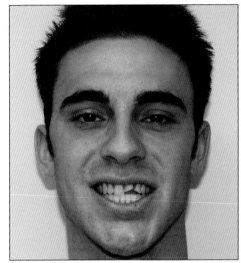

Before

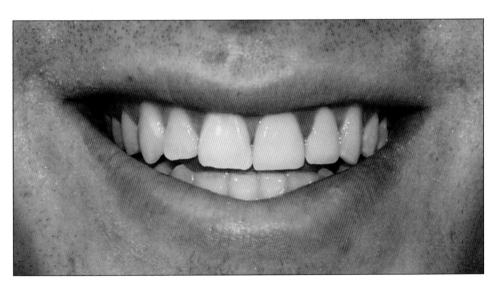

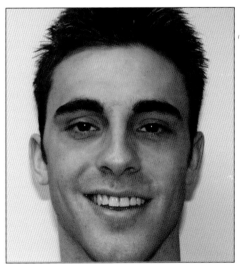

After

But the damage was only temporary. It was easily fixed with two porcelain veneers.

WORN TEETH WITH COLLAPSED BITE

Over the years, grinding of the teeth resulted in their edges being worn away. As the bite collapsed, the aesthetic appearance of the smile was compromised.

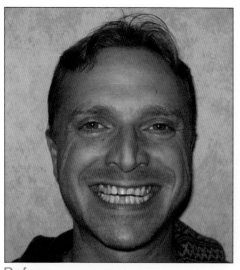

Before

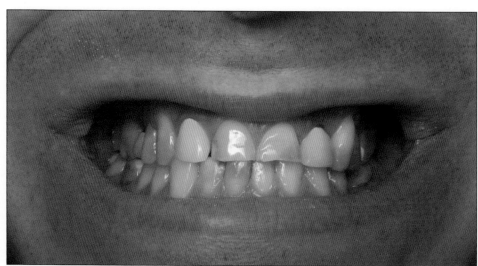

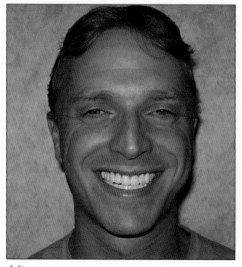

After

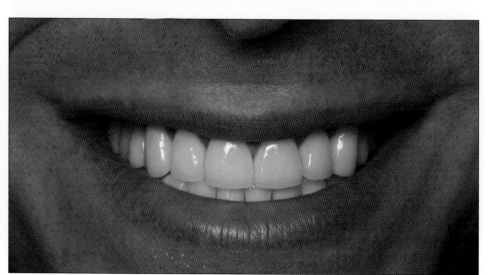

By raising his bite, additional room was created in his mouth.
This allowed his smile to be restored with beautiful all porcelain crowns.

SHORT MAXILLARY LATERAL INCISORS

The short lateral incisors make the two central incisors look too large.
His smile has an unbalanced look.

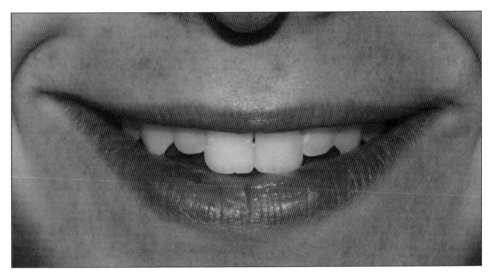
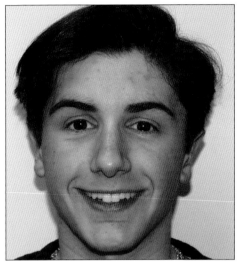

Before

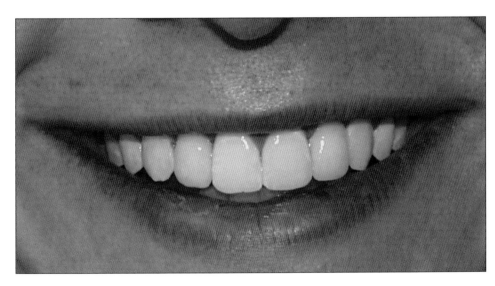
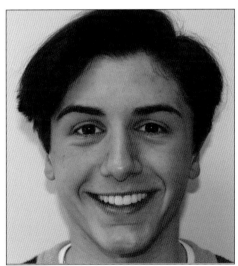

After

By simply adding two porcelain veneers in two visits, he now has a perfect smile
which compliments his face.

AGING SMILE

Here we see how the overall face seems older as a
smile wears and turns yellow.

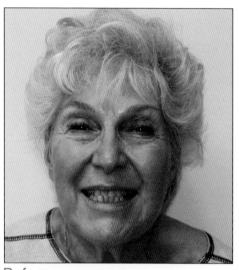

Before

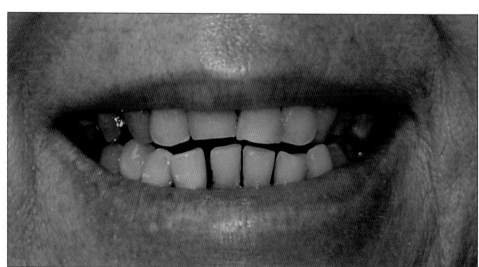

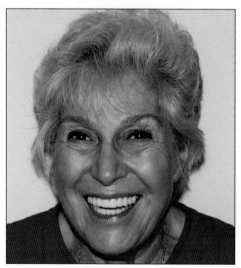

After

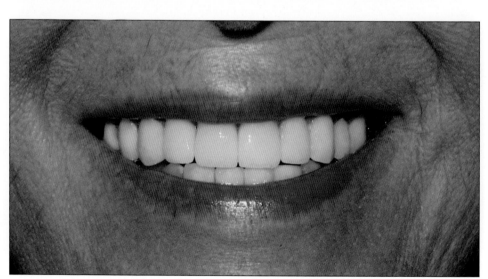

It is truly amazing how fourteen porcelain veneers placed in this mouth in
two visits took ten years off her looks.

MISSING LATERAL INCISORS

This young man was missing his maxillary lateral incisors since birth.
He was very unhappy with all the anterior spaces when he smiled.

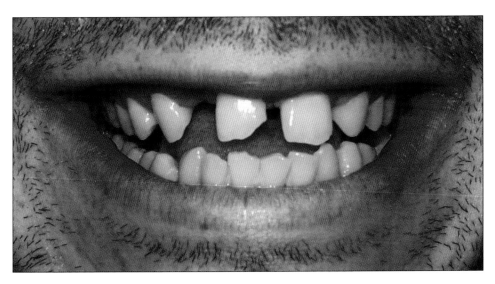
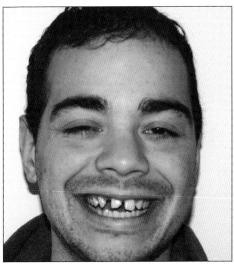

Before

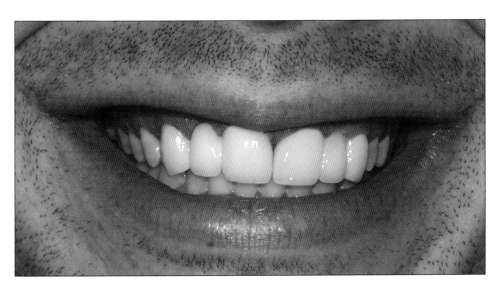
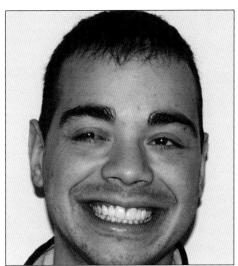

After

Two porcelain bridges were placed which closed the space and allowed him to regain
his confidence when he smiled.

GUM RECESSION AND OLD CROWNS

This is a case of old porcelain-fused-to-metal crowns where the gums have receded due to periodontal disease.

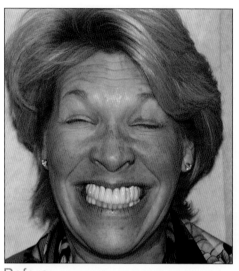

Before

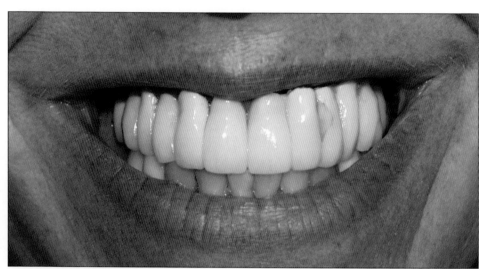

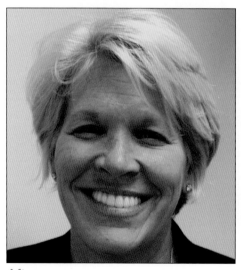

After

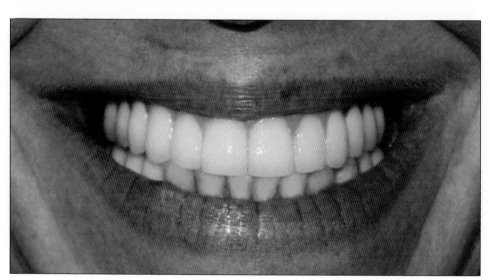

By adding dental implants and using "pink" porcelain gum tissue on top of new porcelain-fused-to-metal crowns, a more natural looking smile was created.

SPACES AROUND LOWER INCISORS

This young woman did not like the spaces around her mandibular incisor teeth.
She wanted the spaces closed as soon as possible.

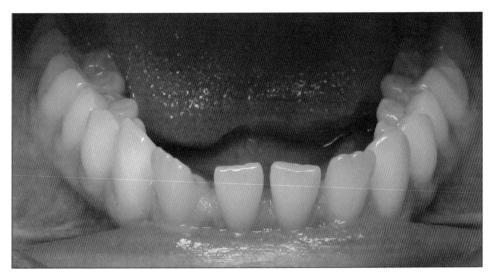

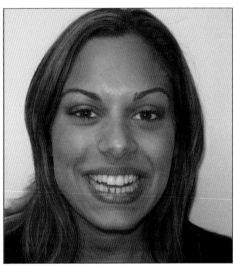

Before

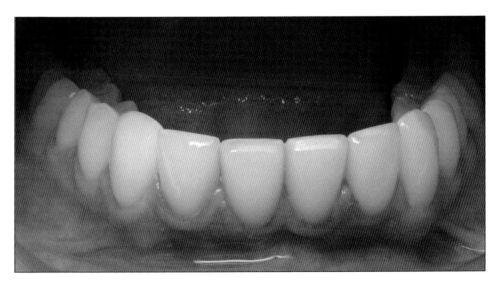

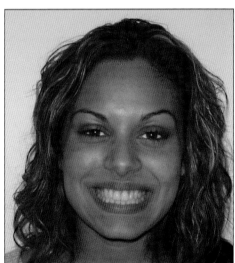

After

Her request was easily granted by placing six porcelain veneers in one week.

ADVANCED GUMMY SMILE

Excessive gums can cause a distortion of the smile.

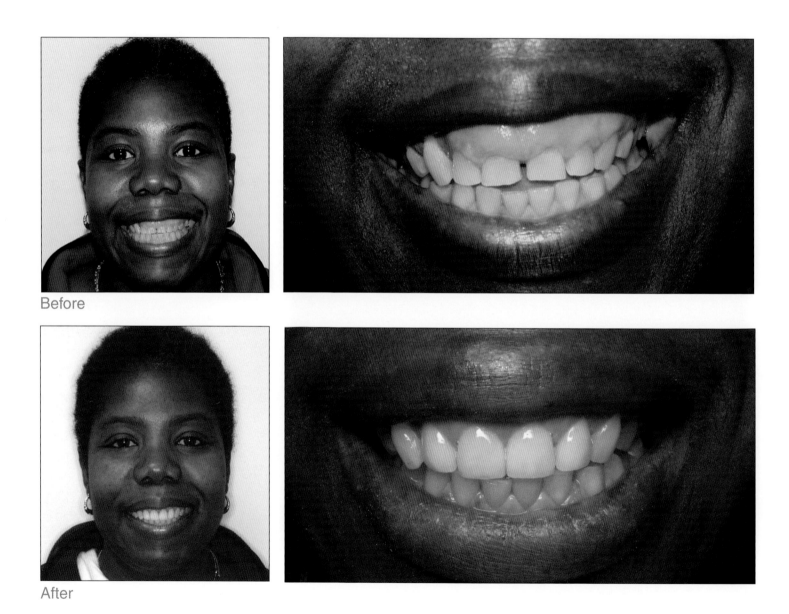

Before

After

The solution here was a surgical gum lift and bone reduction followed
by four porcelain veneers.

DARK TEETH WITH WORN EDGES

Nothing makes a person's face look older than dark teeth with worn biting edges.

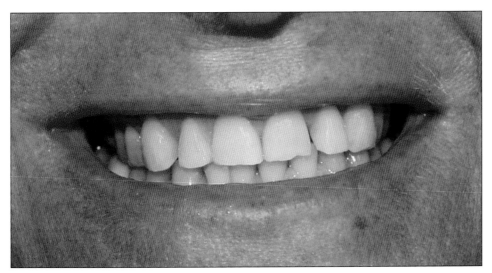

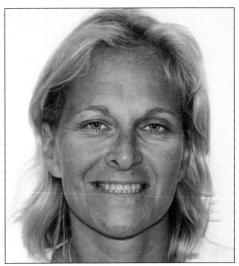

Before

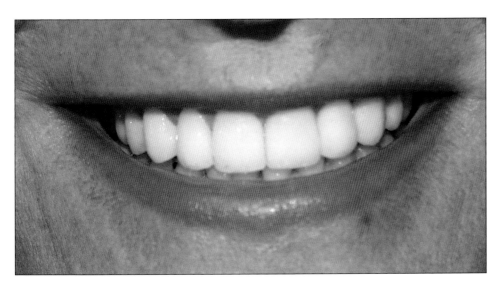

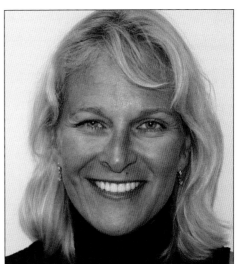

After

A more youthful smile was established with twelve porcelain veneers.

MISSING MANY TEETH AND BITE COLLAPSE

Over a period of time, this gentleman lost many teeth. As teeth were lost,
his bite collapsed and his ability to chew became more difficult.

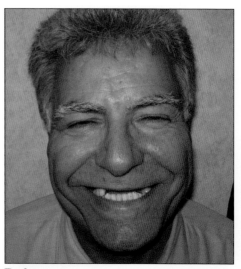

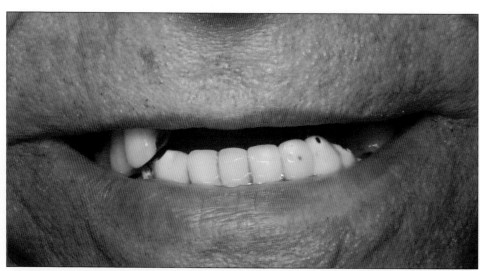

Before

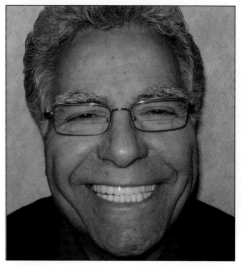

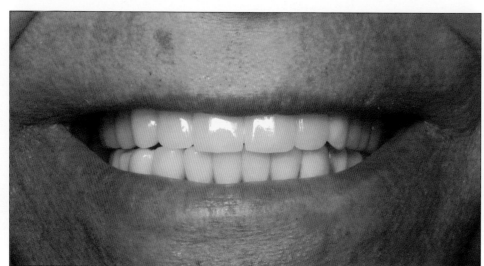

After

Over a period of six months, his mouth was fully restored with a combination of dental
implants and porcelain-fused-to-gold crowns.

WORN EDGES FROM GRINDING

This patient wore down the edges of his teeth over many years.
This contributed to a bite collapse and an unsightly smile.

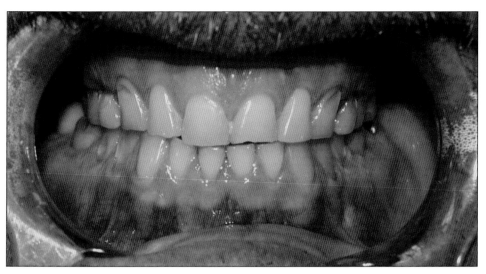
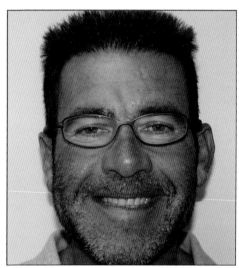

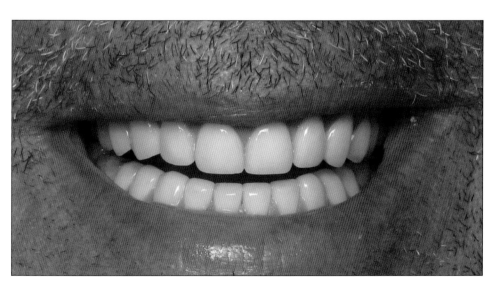
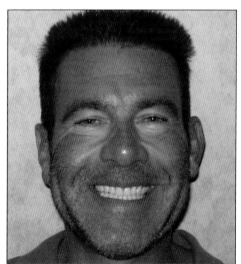

In just a couple of visits, his mouth was restored with a combination of
porcelain crowns and porcelain veneers.

DECALCIFICATIONS

Here we see teeth with decalcifications throughout this patient's mouth.
This made her feel self conscious about her smile.

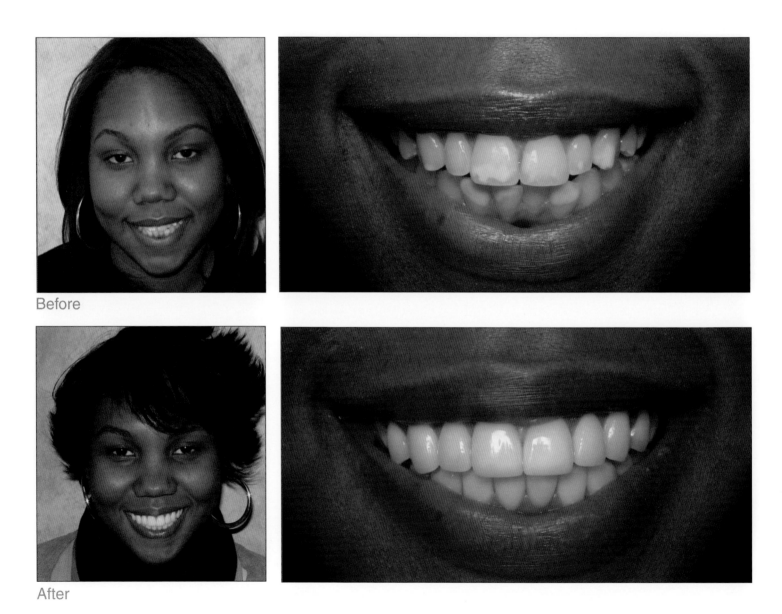

Before

After

With fourteen porcelain veneers placed in two visits, her smile was fully restored.

114

INTRUDED INCISORS

This case would take about two years to correct with orthodontic treatment.

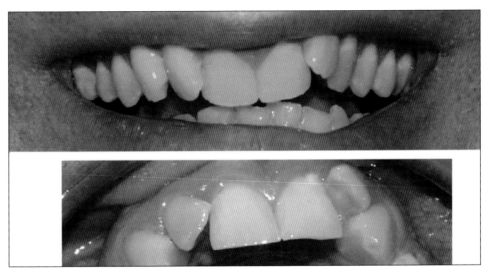
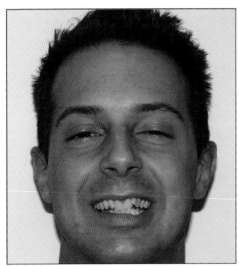

Before

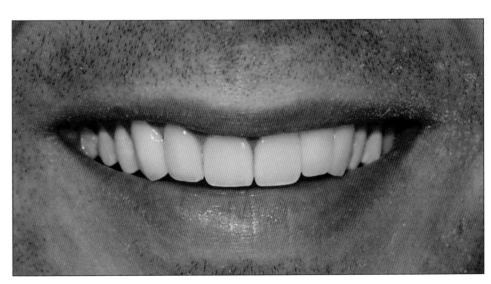
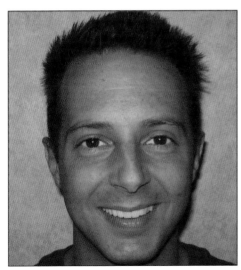

After

Instead, this patient opted for root canal treatment and porcelain veneers in order to correct his smile in just three visits.

SHORT INCISORS AND CROOKED TEETH

A combination of problems contributed to this patient's unattractive smile. He had short incisors, a poor upper left bridge and a constricted upper right side. In addition, his lower teeth were very crooked.

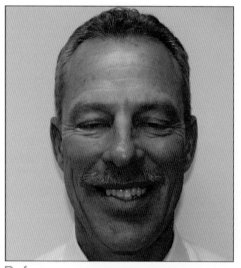
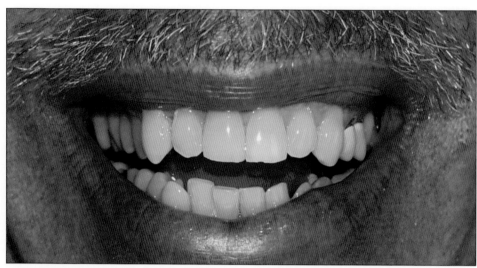

Before

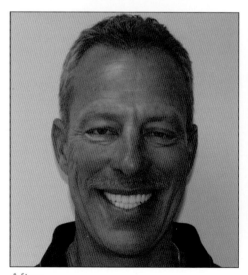
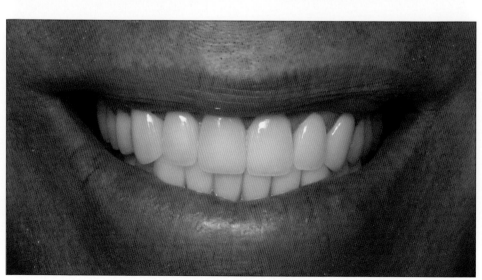

After

This smile makeover was accomplished with a new porcelain bridge and porcelain veneers.

DECAYED CROOKED TEETH

Years of neglect led to advanced breakdown of these crooked teeth.

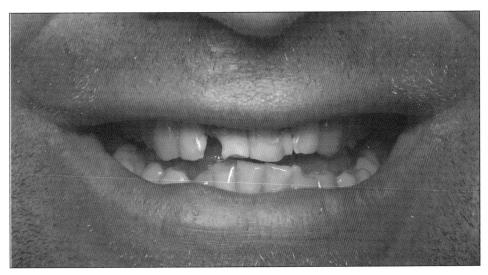
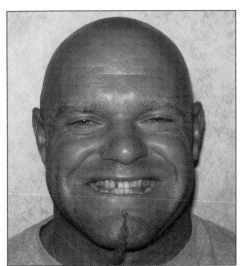

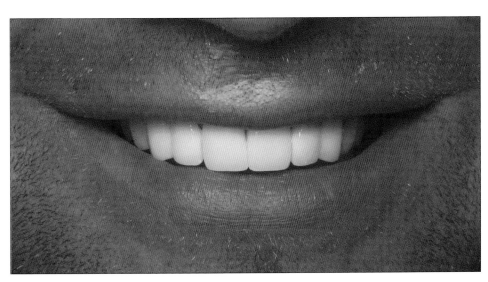
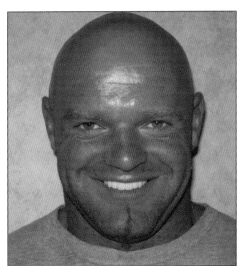

Another porcelain veneer miracle restored this patient's smile in just two visits.

ROOT CANAL STAINED TEETH

This patient's maxillary left central and lateral incisors were stained after blood and decay were left inside her teeth following root canal treatment. Her right lateral incisor had an old bonded restoration.

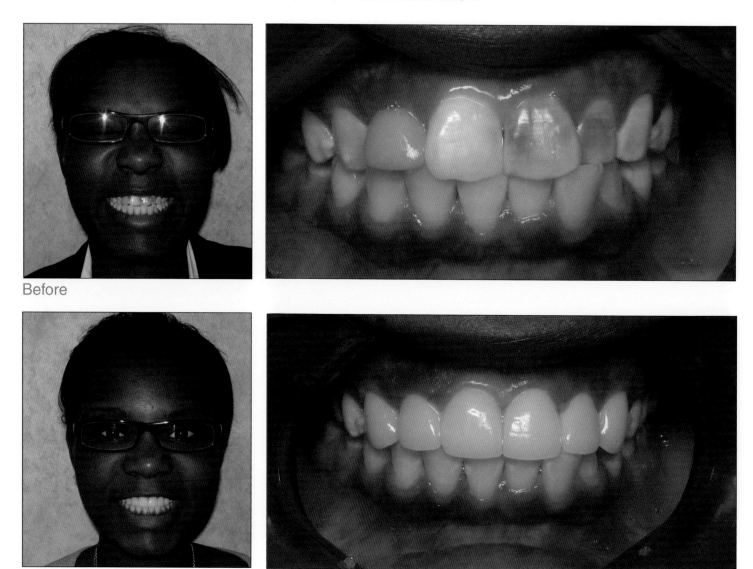

Before

After

In one week, a beautiful smile was restored with the addition of six maxillary veneers.

COSMETIC EFFECTS OF PERIODONTAL DISEASE

Advanced periodontal disease caused severe gum recession and loosening of all his teeth.

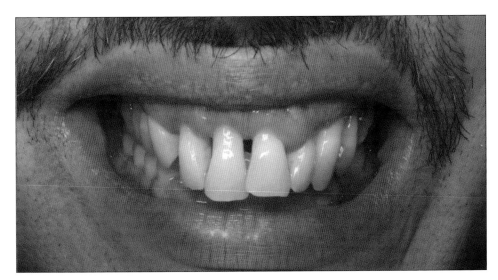
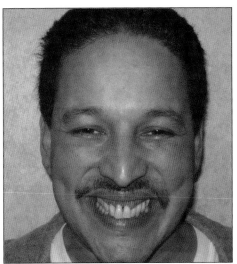

Before

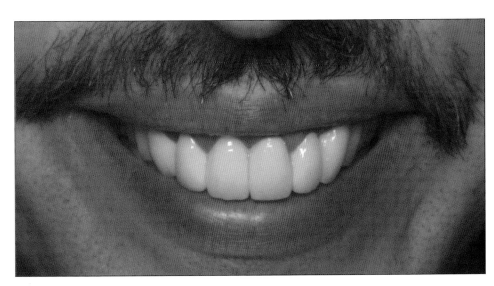
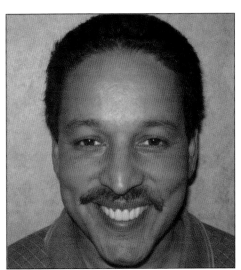

After

After periodontal treatment was completed, his teeth were restored
with porcelain-fused-to-metal-crowns.

VERY CROOKED TEETH

This patient was told that she would need extensive orthodontic treatment.
She wanted an alternative where she could have a cosmetically acceptable mouth
as quickly as possible.

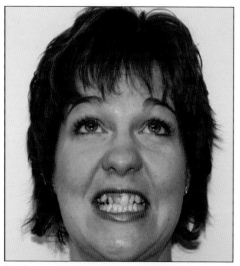

Before

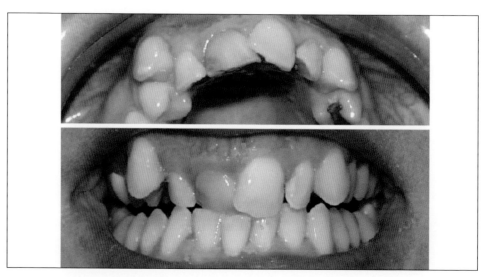

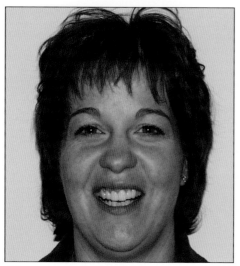

After

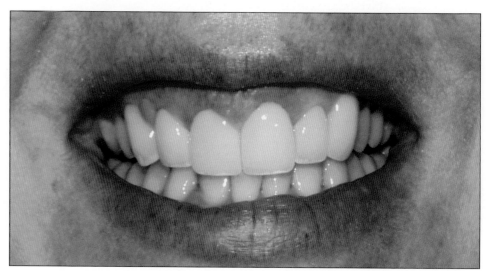

After a minor gum lift surgery, and root canal treatment, she was able to have the
smile she always dreamed of with ten porcelain veneers.

GUM RECESSION AND FLARED TEETH

This patient's teeth flared out thereby increasing her overjet. Her gums receded due to the effects of periodontal disease.

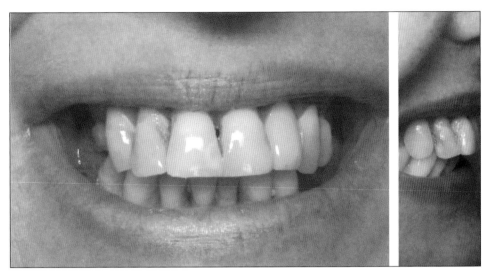
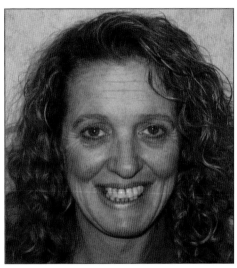

Before

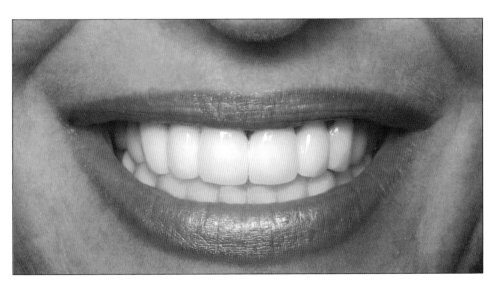
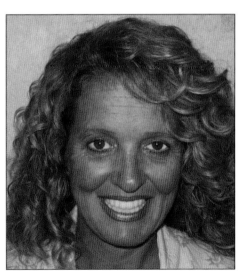

After

After gum treatment for the periodontal disease, her teeth were pulled back and splinted with porcelain-fused-to-gold crowns.

ADVANCED FULL MOUTH RECONSTRUCTION

This patient required a full mouth rehabilitation with root canal treatments, periodontal treatment and full upper and lower splinted porcelain-fused-to-gold crowns.

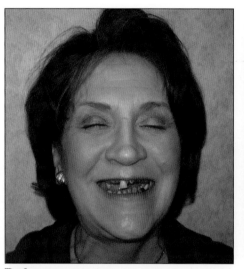
Before

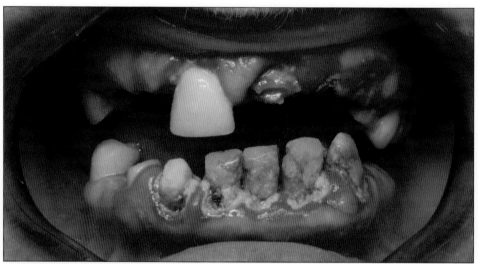

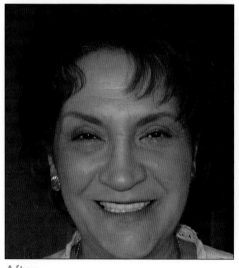
After

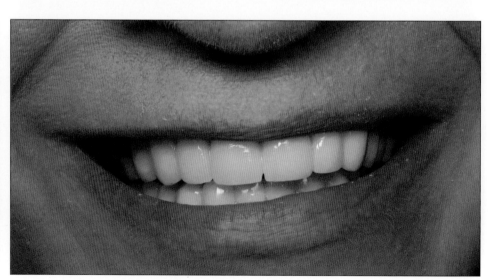

Using techniques available today in modern cosmetic dentistry, even an advanced case such as this one can have such an amazing outcome.

OLD PORCELAIN METAL CROWNS

This patient wanted her opaque and yellow porcelain metal crowns replaced with something more translucent. At the same time, she wanted a whiter smile.

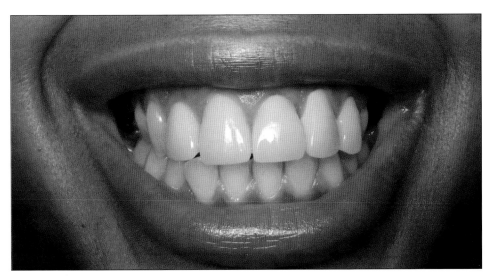
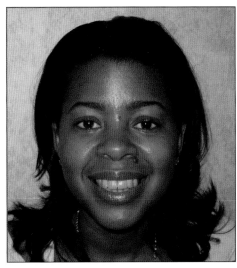

Before

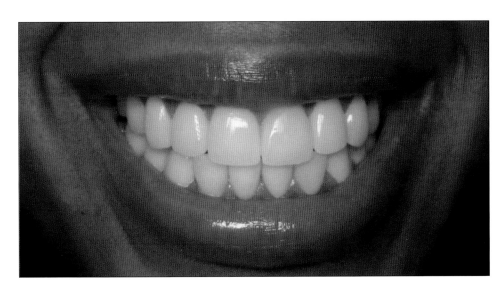
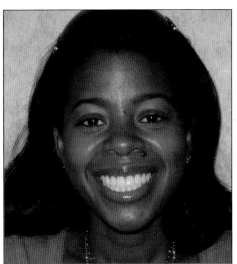

After

The solution was placing all porcelain crowns and porcelain veneers to create that extraordinary white and realistic looking smile.

UNUSUAL IMPACTED CANINE

This is a situation where the maxillary right canine was ankylosed (fused) to the bone and did not erupt. The baby tooth below was still in place. Other teeth in the arch were out of alignment.

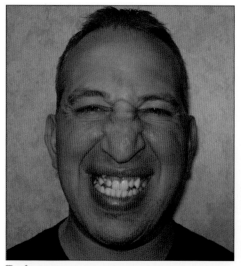 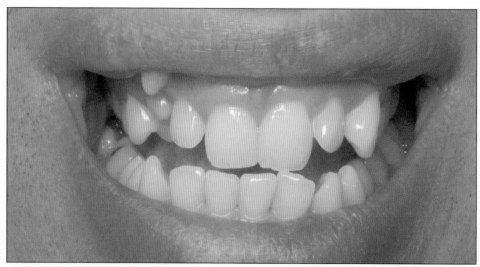

Before

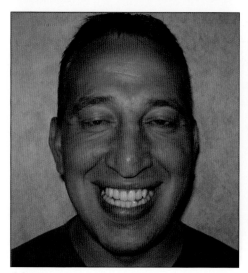 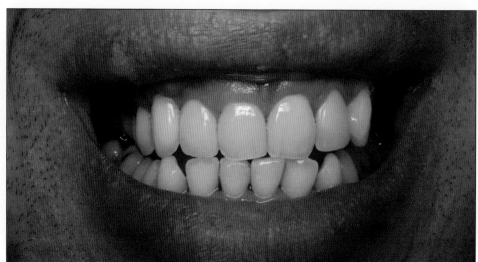

After

To create a pleasing smile, his baby tooth was removed and replaced with a three unit all porcelain bridge. A porcelain veneer was placed on the opposite lateral incisor for balance. Finally, pink bonded composite resin was placed over the tip of the ankylosed canine to camouflage it when he smiled.

WORN YELLOW AND BROWN TEETH

The worn edges and color of this patient's teeth seriously detracted from his smile.

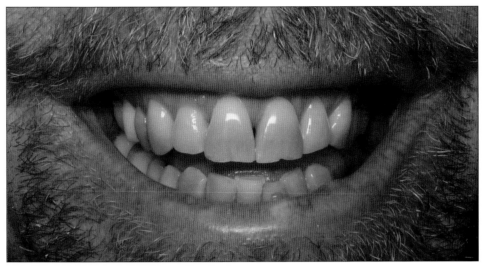
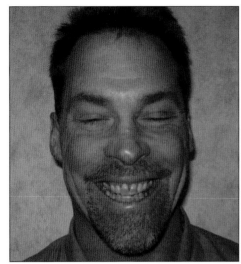

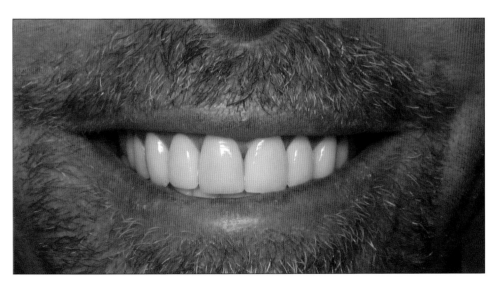
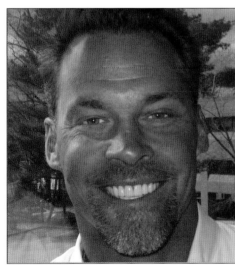

After

A bright and healthy looking smile was quickly established with sixteen porcelain veneers.

GUMMY SMILE WITH SMALL BICUSPIDS

This patient wanted to lessen the gummy smile look and increase the size of her maxillary bicuspids.

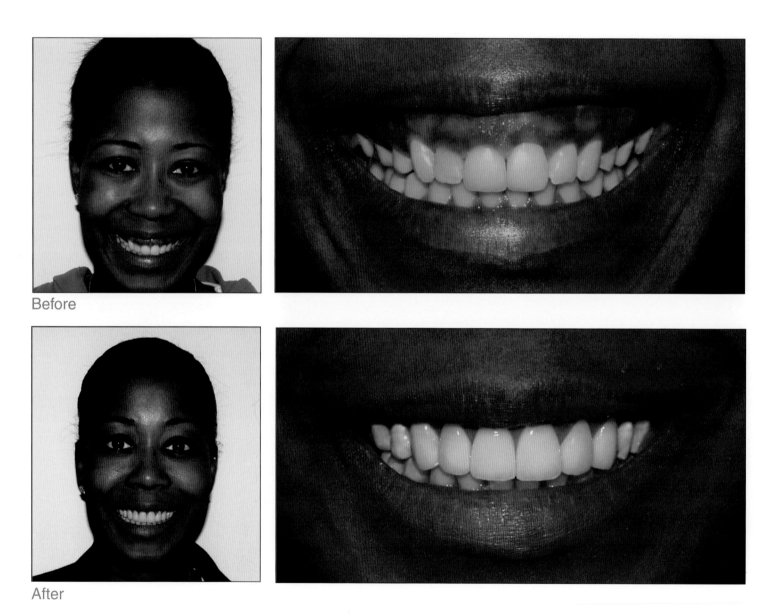

Before

After

The solution was maxillary crown lengthening surgery followed by six porcelain veneers.

ADVANCED DECAY

Even teeth with advanced decay can be saved if the patient is motivated to do so.

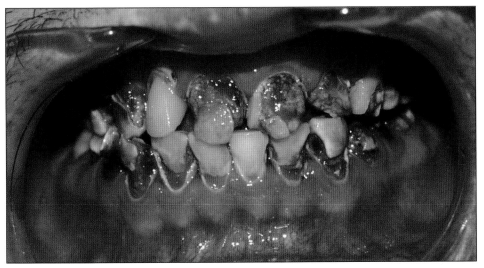
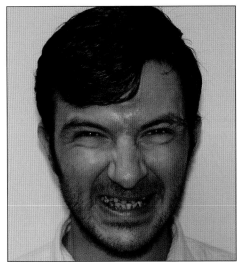

Before

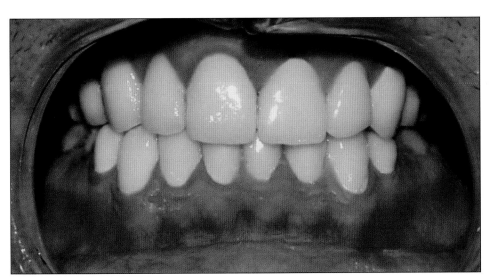
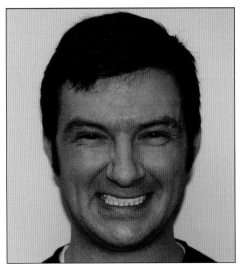

After

After several root canal treatments and treatment for gum disease, porcelain-fused-to-metal crowns were made to re-establish the lost bite and smile.

OVERLAPPING CENTRAL INCISORS

A very common problem is overlapping of the maxillary central incisors.

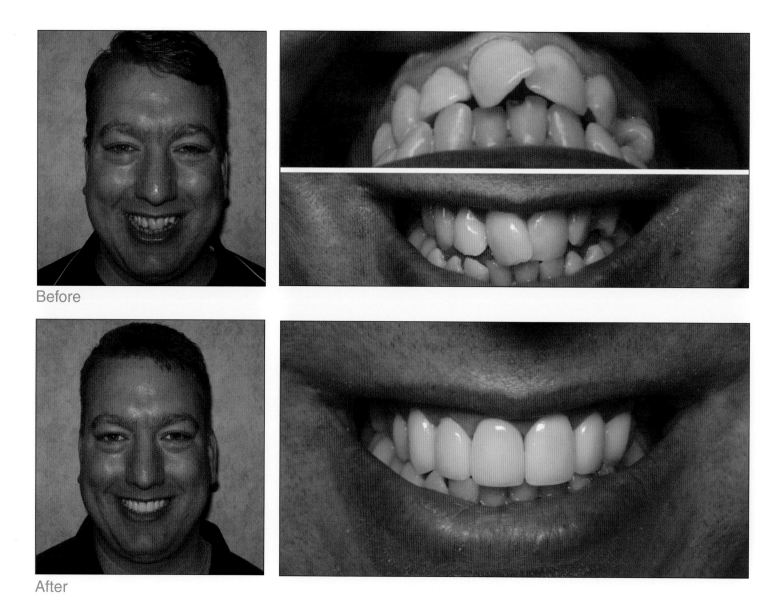

Before

After

This patient avoided long orthodontic treatment by having six porcelain veneers placed over the maxillary anterior teeth.

ANTERIOR CROWDING

Here we see a situation where there is not enough room for his anterior teeth.
He did not want to go through years of orthodontic treatment.

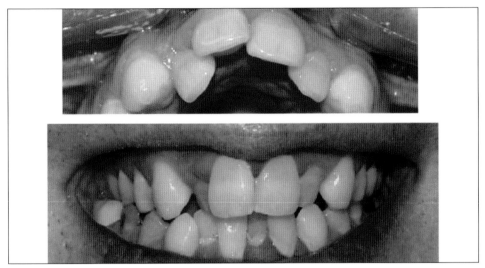

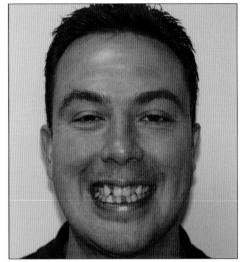

Before

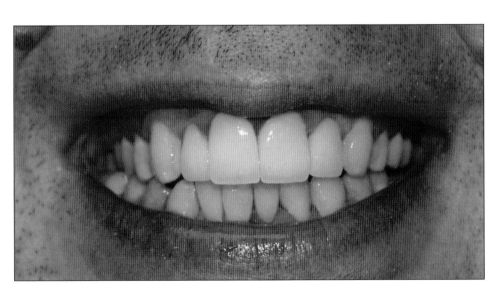

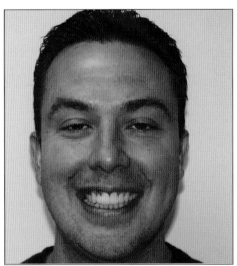

After

His solution was a minor gingivectomy to lower his gums on selected teeth,
two root canal treatments and six porcelain veneers.

TETRACYCLINE STAINED TEETH

This is a case of severe tetracycline stained teeth with worn enamel surfaces.

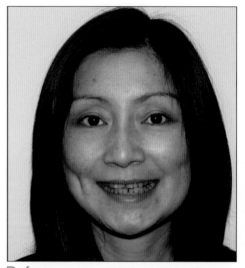

Before

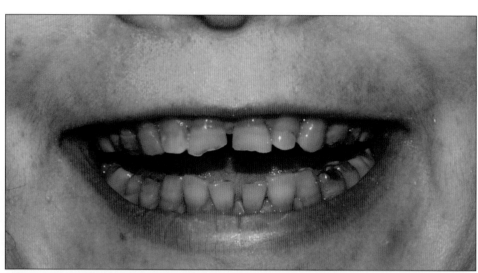

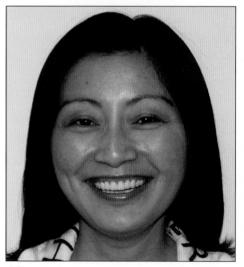

After

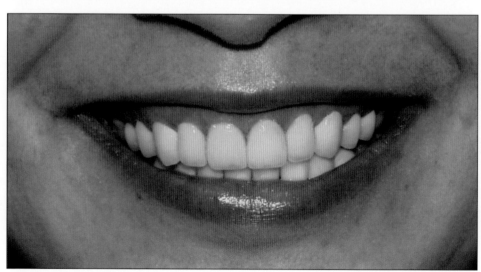

Fortunately, she was able to get a beautiful smile in two visits
with eighteen porcelain veneers.

ANTERIOR OPEN BITE

This young woman had a classic anterior open bite leaving her central incisors flared and pointed outward. She did not want to show any space between her upper and lower teeth when she smiled.

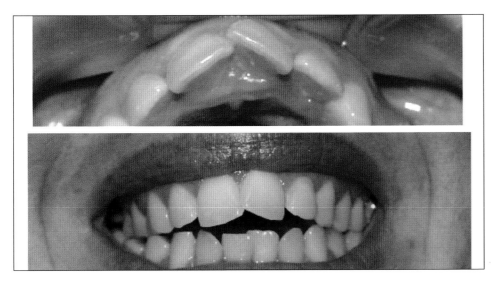
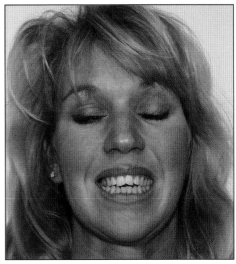

Before

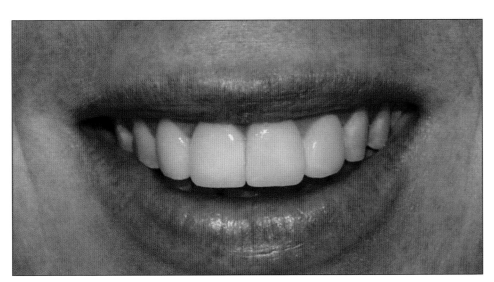
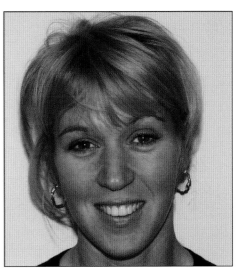

After

Her wish came true with one root canal for alignment purposes and four porcelain veneers. All treatment was completed in three visits.

131

Real People with Cosmetic Dental Problems Tell Their Stories

I could devote this entire book to the wonderful stories about how cosmetic dentistry has changed the lives of thousands of my patients over the past three decades.

However, I think that letting you read some of the letters and emails sent to me from my actual patients in their own words is more powerful than anything I could say.

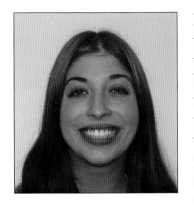

People are constantly telling me how lucky I am to have such naturally, beautiful teeth. Little do they know it's compliments to you, your staff and your wonderful work. Being petrified of visiting dentists and cursed with a low tolerance for pain, I put off having veneers for years. To my amazement the whole procedure from beginning to end was easy and smooth. You not only were professional and gentle, but your humor also served to allay my anxiety. Now, I have the most spectacular teeth and a smile that wins me compliments constantly. I am so happy! My only regret is that I didn't do it sooner.

A.S.

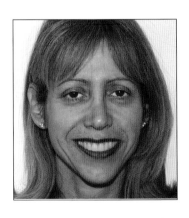

Dear Dr. Kurpis,

It's been two months since I've had the porcelain veneers on my teeth and I wanted to let you know that I am extremely happy with the results. Not only do my teeth look and feel natural, but having a beautiful smile makes me feel great. I have a confident feeling about myself, knowing that I now have an attractive and bright smile. Just today, a stranger complimented me on having such a beautiful smile. People really do notice my smile!

If any prospective clients have concerns or questions about getting porcelain veneers, I would highly recommend they do it. Thanks for doing a great job!

Sincerely,
B.Z.

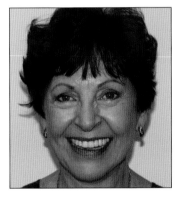

Dear Dr. Kurpis,
People always used to tell me I had a beautiful smile. When they stopped mentioning it, I realized I needed help. My teeth had turned yellow and streaked in my 70 years. I researched several cosmetic dentistry procedures. You were the most professional and the best informed as to my needs. I appreciated how you painstakingly prepared my teeth, advising me of each step, and applied porcelain laminates in a perfect shade to my upper teeth-without any pain! I smile now with confidence and, though the lines in my face weren't removed, people won't believe my age, as my teeth look 50 years younger.

C.C.

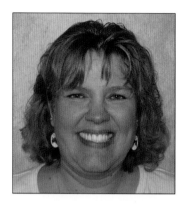

Dear Dr. Kurpis,

At the age of 45, I was sure my life was over. I was not a fan of dentists, (having many bad experiences in the past) and let's face it, most people are not, being afraid of pain and the money issues the way that they are today.

I went onto your web site and for the first time in my life, I had a glimmer of hope, thinking that maybe you would be able to help me. I called and made an appointment with Gretchen, who made me feel really comfortable by telling me that you were indeed the person who could help me. I walked into your office depressed and feeling alone. We discussed options, pricing and loan options and I walked out of your office with a new hope and a new life to look forward to, all to be completed in a matter of months.

I have to be honest that although there was a light at the end of the tunnel, I was scared of the pain and discomfort that I would have to bear. With each procedure and visit that I had, you and your staff were awesome. The pride that you take in your work that you do, and the way that the girls work as a team, made being a patient of yours so much easier. Not one procedure caused me pain and I did not dread going to my appointments.

Here it is, five months later and I will never forget the office visit when you handed me the mirror and I saw the "new me" for the first time. The tears of joy ran down my face and I saw the pride on your face! Not once did I ever feel that I was just another patient. Now, every day when I look in the mirror, I see a beautiful smile and when I go out, other people do too and tell me so.

You truly have a gift and I am so glad that I found you. Thank you for being you.

Sincerely,

D.M.

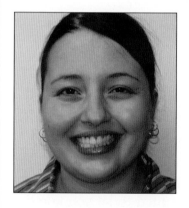

I just want to thank you, Dr. Kurpis, for giving me a reason to smile again. Before all these procedures I was very unhappy with my smile. Everytime I used to talk to people I would look the other way so they would not see my teeth. I hated pictures and would never smile. I always said to myself, I have to fix this problem so I went to you, MY HERO! Now I talk to people face to face without turning away and I smile often.

Thank you Dr. Kurpis,

D.M.

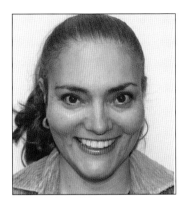

Thank you Dr. Kurpis for a beautiful smile. For several months I searched the web for a cosmetic dentist who could design a smile that would complement my facial features. Only your Website offered the kind of natural looking smile that I was looking for. Most other websites showed before and after photos that had a very "one size fits all" look that did not appear very natural at all. I also found your credentials to be the very best I could find. You are clearly the most qualified expert in your field with a very talented eye for aesthetics. In two visits you were able to transform my widely gapped teeth into a beautiful natural smile that truly reflects my personality. I look younger, healthier, and much happier. Simply put, Dr. Kurpis, you are the very best.

Sincerely,

E.K.

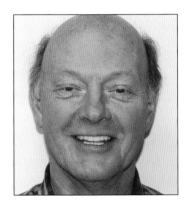

Greetings Dr. Kurpis,

I've been meaning to write you ever since you completed the work on me. I can't tell you how delighted I am with my new smile. I was out in Hollywood last week and one of the producers asked me to star in his movie. I told him I couldn't because I was just made president of my multi-million dollar company. My wife brings me my slippers and the paper everyday now when I come home from work all because of my new smile! NOT REALLY- - but one thing is true! I AM DELIGHTED because for the first time that I can remember I can really smile again! I look at pictures of myself from the past and I can see everyone else in the picture has teeth showing, but there I am-tight lipped. What a difference now! Every once in a while I still catch myself holding back a toothy grin, out of shame, and then I remember my smile is no longer a negative but a huge positive.

I also have to tell you how impressed I was with Francy and the girls at the desk. They made my two visits very pleasant. They were so pleasant and very professional.

I'm amazed that you could do all of that extensive work and yet I never had a problem with any pain or real discomfort. Even the temporaries fit well and were more than adequate for the two weeks that I had them. After the procedure I expected to have some problems with sensitivity or adjusting to my new bite, especially since you lengthened my front teeth a little. There was none of that. My final caps and jackets look extremely natural and they fit the gum line perfectly. Even when I floss, the floss fits just right between the spacing of my teeth. The whiteness that we chose is exactly what I had hoped for. The results just couldn't be any better in my opinion!

I put my full faith and trust in you and I was not disappointed.

Sincerely,

G.K.

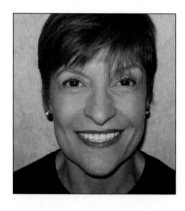

Dear Dr. Kurpis,

Just a quick note to say my "grillwork" looks great. Thank you again. In fact, they got to unexpectedly be on air that night! I did an interview for WEEK-END TODAY on of all things...Bill Clinton "unhappily" turning 60. I'm getting a copy of the segment and putting it on our website so you can refer potential clients to a happy, smiling person.

Warmest regards,

J.S.

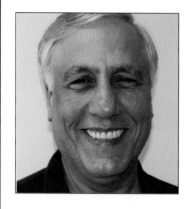

Dear Dr. Kurpis,

Thanks so much for restoring my smile. As far as my implants are concerned, I cannot tell the difference between these and my natural teeth. I can chew anything with confidence again.

I cannot thank you enough.

Regards,

J.A.

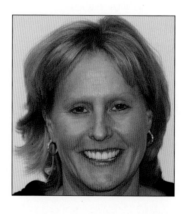

My experience and thoughts on my veneers.

My teeth have never been my best attribute, and I have always been self-conscious of the way they looked in addition to envying those with nice teeth. I struggled with my decision to spend this kind of money on my teeth, but finally decided to visit Dr. Kurpis' office based on extensive research I did on the Internet to find an expert in the field.

I visited the Ridgewood office in early September of 2002, which I traveled an hour each way. Dr. Kurpis and I discussed many options, as well as cost options. On my first visit, I made the decision to "just do it", and I am glad I did. I took a loan out on my 401K which I can pay back interest free. An option one might want to visit.

I had my first appointment in early October, and I had 16 teeth worked on. I left the office that day with 16 temporaries. I was scheduled to come back in later October, and when I left the office that day, I left with my permanent 16 new veneers. I felt like a new person. I felt more confident, I felt pretty, I felt and looked great. On a few occasions since then, on meeting a person whom I had never met prior, they mentioned what a nice smile I had. Something I had never in my life experienced. I am at this point re-doing all my other teeth, the ones that are not as visible. I am doing a few a year, which my insurance covers at some percentage. I was in Dr. Kurpis' office the other day for a cleaning, and he asked me "How are you doing with your veneers?" I said, "It was the best thing I ever did, other than quit smoking." That is pretty powerful. I think about it, and I had wished I had done this many years earlier. All the years of not feeling my best, and not having the confidence that I have now. I always knew that when I meet someone, or am talking to someone with bad teeth, it leaves and undesirable impression in my mind. I knew that I had left that same impression on others when I spoke with them. Not a good feeling. I am one person who is very happy that I made the decision to have a beautiful smile.

Sincerely,

T.C.

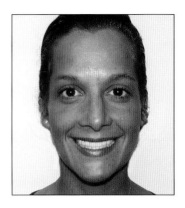

Hi Dr. Kurpis:

I want to thank you from the bottom of my heart for helping me change my appearance and in turn changing my life.

I was afraid and ashamed for years to even go to a dentist because of the extensive damage to my teeth. I walked into your office for a consult and walked out feeling more hopeful than ever before.

I took the plunge 2 years ago and haven't looked back since. I have a great new job that depends on my confidence and professional appearance. Without my radiant smile I doubt I would have been able to do this. I was afraid to have work done because of how much it was going to cost but even that was easy to work out.

It's been two years and I haven't had any problems with my teeth. I work in the medical field and I've even had other dentists comment on what great teeth I have. (No one realizes half the time that they're veneers). I recommend that anyone even thinking about cosmetic dentistry "just do it"- you owe it to yourself to feel good. Take the first step and I promise you won't regret it.

Your grateful patient,

G.M.

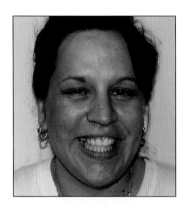

Dr. Kurpis,

I am writing this letter to thank you for my new smile. I still can't beleive it. I had bonding on my two front teeth for 13 years due to a huge gap in my front teeth.

At the time I thought that bonding was an easy way to fix my appearance. I was just happy the gap was gone.

Well the day I got the bonding I realized the teeth were too thick and overlapping the original teeth to cover the gap. I then started to have a hard time pronouncing certain letters. I also had a very bucked-tooth appearance. For years I had kept my mouth closed and never smiled, especially in pictures. I have been very self-conscious about my smile and could not stand my appearance. Then I heard about veneers, a new process to fix gaps with a thin porcelain material. I can tell you I was very skeptical due to my last dental experience. Doing my teeth over was a big step for me.

My first experience at your office was very professional staff was great (thank you Gretchen!), who made me feel very comfortable. She explained the procedure and let me view the actual veneers. When my veneers were ready she reviewed them with me. They were ready in only eight days. In the patient time however, it was a very nervous time for me. I wondered if I did the right thing. Once you put the actual veneers in my mouth, I was shocked at the difference it made. I could not believe it. It has been two weeks and I love my teeth more and more every day. Thank you very much for my new smile. I definitely would recommend you to my friends and already have two co-workers who say they looked beautiful. Actually, people can't take it any more because I keep talking about them. Well like I said to everyone, you are the best! Thank you again.

J.O.

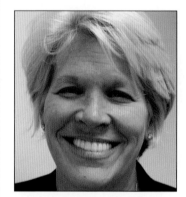

J.E.

Dr. Kurpis is a genius! I never thought the implant experience could be so painless. My teeth look gorgeous, I'm not afraid to smile and my family says I look much happier all the time. Kudos to Dr. Kurpis and his entire staff.

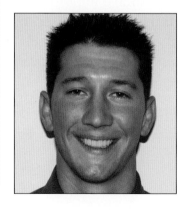

I would like to offer a word of advice to anyone with even the littlest bit of interest in cosmetic dentistry. Before I had my teeth fixed I was a bit skeptical, and so were those around me. Since having it done all minds have changed. I smile all day long, and the people around me can see the difference. It is something I wanted done for a long time but was searching for the right doctor. Believe me when I tell you, "you have come to the right place." At my consultation Dr. Kurpis made me a promise that I would love my new smile. Today I can say thank you because I am like a new person. Like I said earlier, if you are even slightly interested then get it done. My confidence level is sky-high. It has truly changed my life.

J.B.

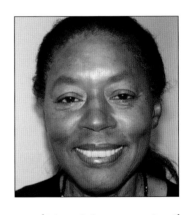

Dr. Kurpis,

 Major dental work suggesting caps, implants, or other irreversible changes to your mouth can seem unduly unsettling.

However, an examination of the pros and cons can result in giving your teeth what they need. With excellent dental care I have been given a spectacular and lasting smile, and a mouth that feels smooth and silky with the added benefit of improving my overall health.

L.R.S.

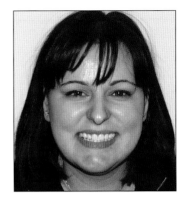

Hi Dr. Kurpis,

I wanted to take the time to thank you again for the beautiful work that you did on my teeth. My whole life, I have had many troubles with my teeth. I have gone through many minor surgeries and spent a good four years wearing braces. Even with all of the dental work that I had done, I was far from happy with my smile.

I dreaded taking pictures. I was even too self conscious to smile at people at home, not to mention people that I met on the streets and at work, and many people viewed me as being unfriendly.

I am so fortunate to have come across your web site that day. It gave me such hope that maybe I could have a wonderful smile too. I called and made my appointment and from the first time I met with you, I felt so comfortable. It's been very difficult to visit a dentist since I have had so many dreadful experiences. I was afraid that I was getting my hopes up and never believed that I could afford something like this. I walked out of your office that day glowing. I was so excited knowing that in a few days, I was going to have a perfect smile.

Throughout this past year, I have smiled so much and you can really notice the difference in my personality. My nickname at work now is "Smiley".

139

There doesn't go a day that I don't get a compliment or hear how beautiful my smile is. Nobody can tell that I have veneers. You do an amazing job and it looks 100% natural. I am so grateful to have met you and to have chosen you to be my smile savior.

Thank you so much for changing my life. Thank you for helping me. My confidence is high. My self esteem is high. My smile is beautiful and I owe it all to you.

M.M.

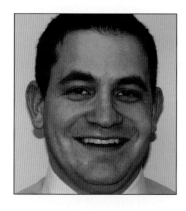

Dear Dr. Kurpis:

Thank you very much for all of the work you have done on my teeth. Both you and your staff have treated me well and your quality of work was fantastic. Having Dr. Kurpis put porcelain veneers on my teeth is one of the best decisions I could have made. As a young attorney, my image is very important to me. Not only was Dr. Kurpis' quality of work fantastic, but dealing with him and his staff was a joy as well. They made a potentially complicated procedure very simple and an enjoyable experience. I highly recommend Dr. Kurpis to anyone who needs any type of cosmetic dental work.

Sincerely,

M.S.

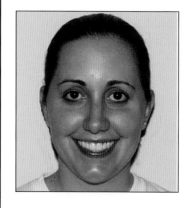

With my wedding only three months away, I knew I was not happy with my smile and I wanted everything to be perfect for this special day in my life. I had braces as a kid but my teeth had shifted over the years and whitening procedures were not giving me the results that I was looking for. You explained to me how veneers could give me a perfect smile that I was never able to achieve. I was nervous to schedule the procedure because you only get one set of permanent teeth so you need to be careful what you do with them! You and your staff erased all of my concerns so I went ahead and booked the procedure. It's been one week since the procedure and I am very happy with the results. My smile finally is the way I always envisioned it to be. I can't wait to take my wedding pictures now!

M.L.

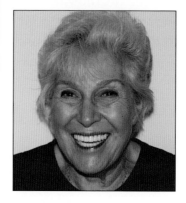

Dear Dr. Kurpis:

Last week you finished my veneers, and I want you to know how very happy you made me. I used to daydream about teeth like these-and now I have them!

What's completely amazing is that you not only gave me beautiful, real-looking "new" teeth so quickly, but in so doing you also fixed my poor bite-and gave my mouth, smile, and entire face a refreshing new look! I absolutely love it! (So does everyone who sees me!) The result is a wonderful, new, happy attitude about myself and my forthcoming retirement. Dr. Kurpis, with my new look, you have actually "made" that next stage of my life. Thank you so much!

Sincerely,

R.J.

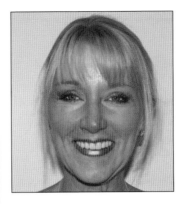

Dear Dr. Kurpis,

About a year ago I had my teeth veneered at your practice. I wanted to tell you that I have been in the entertainment industry for 30 years and yes due to the fact I work on camera have had my share of plastic surgery. Of all of the maintenance I've chosen for myself over the years having my teeth veneered was the BEST decision I ever made. The first thing anyone notices is your teeth! It is the window of your smile and beauty. When you have had bad teeth your confidence slips. My teeth were never extremely terrible but I felt self-conscious because of yellowing. I've tried EVERY product out there. They will never even come close to the result I got with your procedure. So for anyone wondering what to do about their teeth they should definitely consider your veneer procedure.

Thank you.

M.M.

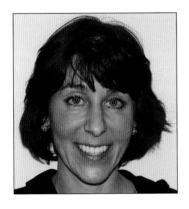

After being involved in a motor vehicle accident in 1997, my teeth were repaired by another dentist with porcelain veneers. The veneers appeared bulky and masculine and fell off frequently. After extreme frustration I was referred to Dr. Kurpis and my mouth was transformed. The veneers fit my mouth better and look perfect. In fact, other dentists have commented that they were unsure if my teeth were veneers because they look so natural. In addition, Dr. Kurpis has a gentle disposition with a great bedside manner. But, most important to me is that my teeth finally stay in my mouth!

M.H.

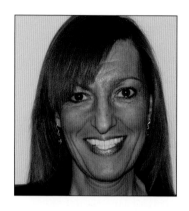

Dear Dr. Kurpis,

It has been just about a year since you did my porcelain veneers. I am still amazed at the difference it has made in my life. My smile was something I was always embarrassed about and wanted to hide.

I had thought many times over the years of doing something about straightening my teeth, but the prospect of wearing braces for several years was not something I could imagine doing. Even with braces I would not have gotten the dramatic effect that the veneers achieved. My teeth are now perfectly straight and whiter than I could have ever imagined. After years and years of the embarrassment I felt due to my crooked smile the dramatic change was accomplished in two visits and over a few short weeks.

Over the past year I have taken on a sales position at my job and this entails traveling to new and existing customers as well as to different conferences and trade shows. My new smile has given me much more confidence when meeting people for the first time. This has helped me tremendously in the way I communicate with clients, colleagues, and in day-to-day life.

I owe this change to my smile makeover. I do have one regret that I think about quite often. That is that I did not have this procedure done many years earlier. This would have made a huge difference in my life in so many ways.

Again, I would like to thank Dr. Kurpis and his friendly staff for doing a great job and for making a dream come true. The dream of having a smile that I use to envy and that I can be proud of. Now I can smile and laugh with confidence and I will always be amazed at the beautiful job that you have done.

With Gratitude and Kind Regards,

M.A.V.

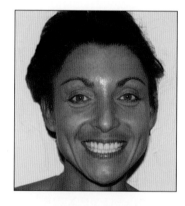

Dear Dr. Kurpis,

Thank you so very much for the fantastic job you have done with my teeth. In the past, I would have smiled on very rare occasions. When I did smile, it was a very smug, closed mouth insincere looking smile. This was due to the fact that I was very embarrassed to smile. I had very crooked, yellow stained teeth, and was very self-conscious. People perceived me as being much too serious or snobby. This was not the case at all.

Since the beautiful job you have done on my teeth, I have been receiving compliments on my smile and my teeth continuously. I wish I would have known about your work years ago. I had never imagined the entire procedure would be so quick and so painless.

Thank you Dr. Kurpis.

Sincerely,

M.K.

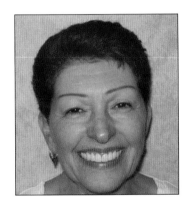

Dear Dr. Kurpis,

Thank you so much for the beautiful new smile. I never thought my teeth could look so good. Not only do my teeth look great, but they are straight and give me so much more confidence when talking. I am so happy you gave me such good advice on correcting not only crooked, but such discolored teeth. My teeth not only look wonderful, but also feel so much better. I will be happy to recommend you to anyone interested in having the best possible smile in such a short time. Your office staff is also very comforting and encouraging. Thank you for making this experience so rewarding.

Regards,

L.E.

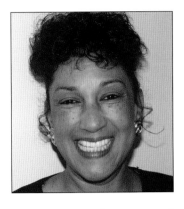

When I decided that I wanted to try dental implants, I wanted the best dentist to do the work, so I went to Dr. Albert Kurpis. Although I thought I would shy away from the cost of the implants, after a thorough explanation on the implant process, assessment of my specific needs, and answers to every question that I asked, I decided to go for it.

Dr. Kurpis' kind and professional manner, and his professional staff really made me feel comfortable. What really sold me on having Dr. Kurpis do my implant procedure was this: I already had bridgework done and he explained how I needed a new bridge along with implants. Again, I was not too happy about the costs. However, he said to me: "what level of quality do you want for your bridgework and implants?" He continued by saying, "right now, your bridgework is equivalent to a Ford. I can give you quality work equivalent to a Rolls Royce." After seeing his numerous certificates in dental and implant surgery, his prominent positions in the American Academy of Implant Dentistry, and knowing that I wanted the best, I had him do the work. I have been very pleased so far with my implants, and I do feel he was the right choice for me. I would not hesitate to recommend him to others seeking implants.

R.B.

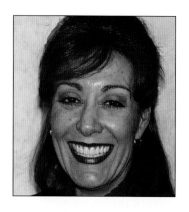

Dear Dr. Kurpis:

They say a picture is worth a thousand words. Perhaps in this case it's not a picture, but a woman's smile and in this particular case the woman's smile is mine.

I wanted to take this opportunity to thank you for not only enhancing the way I look, but also changing the way I feel.

I recently was involved in a photo shoot where the photographer kept echoing what a beautiful smile I had and how it seemed to light my entire face.

That light, or halo of happiness, comes from a talented dentist and a woman who has a reason to smile.

My sincerest thanks,

L.C.

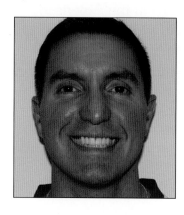

My original dentist suggested I get six crowns. I was very apprehensive about crowns and their cost. Dr. Kurpis explained veneers would be safer, a much healthier alternative, and also, less expensive. Most importantly, he explained that I would love my new smile. HE COULD NOT HAVE BEEN MORE RIGHT!!!

The procedure was painless and only required two visits. The crooked and discolored smile I'd lived with for 40 years was gone forever. My teeth are white, straight, and great looking. I enjoy smiling now and am no longer self-conscious about my smile…instead, I like to show it off. My brother tells me every few weeks: "It's the best investment you've ever made." I couldn't agree more!!!

M.A.

Dear Dr. Kurpis

I just wanted to say thanks for giving me my confidence back! You are truly an artist as well as a great dentist. When I left your office today, I don't think that it was my new teeth that I wasn't used to, per say, I think it was all the attention I was getting---that's hard getting used to! But I love it!

Thank you again,

L.S.

Hi Dr. Kurpis,

This letter is a long time coming, but I have thought about how I would write it everyday since I received my new smile! Since I was a young girl, I have had horrible results and experiences with dentists. I would go to one and they would redo the job, only to have 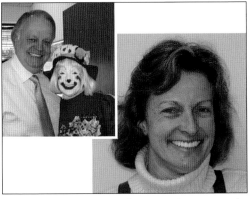 more fall apart. I was never happy with my teeth. Then, in my 30's, I became a clown, a white-face clown. Now I really had to be careful. I taught myself to smile a crooked smile to only show the teeth that were decent and when my party moms would take a picture, I never smiled with my teeth showing. I didn't want to ruin their picture. My Mom had great difficulty with her teeth all her life, but never went to a dentist. When she died, we realized how few pictures we had of her because she did not want her mouth to be photographed.

Then I found you. Just when another doctor was placing "flippers" and suggesting the possibility of dentures, I had to try just one more dentist. That was you and your team! In less than a year, I had implants, bridges and veneers in place and a whole new me!! It actually took me a lot of work to learn to smile again, but I do it ALL the time. I have never had such a beautiful smile in my whole life! Everywhere I go, people make comments about my teeth and how beautiful my smile is! Even when I went to the McDonald's drive-up, the young man said, "I hope you don't mind me saying, but you have

a beautiful smile"! WOW! It is not that easy for a white face clown to have a beautiful smile against all that white make up. But I do, thanks to you. Like an artist, you gave me something that I only dreamed about. I am reminded of how lucky I am and I really appreciate what a fantastic dentist can do. THAT'S YOU!! I just commissioned someone to make a caricature of my clown, Daisy for use in stickers to hand out to kids. When we first saw the rough draft, all my family and friends said "You can't use that one, you can't see your smile. You're always smiling!" So we had to have him redo the picture and add in the smile.

Every time I smile I will think of you and appreciate it all. Hey, if you ever need a clown, you've got one here who is always smiling!! Thanks just doesn't seem like enough.

Yours with a smile,

E.D.V.

Frequently Asked Questions about Different Cosmetic Dentistry Procedures.

Before proceeding with cosmetic dental procedures that will change your smile, there may be questions you need answered. Be sure to ask these questions to your cosmetic dentist so that there are no misunderstandings. If you are uncomfortable with the answer you hear, either do not do the procedure or go for a second opinion. Sometimes several opinions are necessary to give you the peace of mind to go ahead with changes to your smile. Whatever it takes, become well informed and do not let doubt become a barrier to a great looking smile.

I have received numerous questions about different procedures over the years. Here are a few samples of questions people most frequently have asked when inquiring about cosmetic dental procedures. These questions are organized into five groups of the most popular cosmetic dental procedures.

Porcelain Veneers

Teeth Whitening and Bleaching

Dental Implants

Caps, Crowns, Inlays, and Fixed Bridges

Removable Bridges and Dentures

Porcelain Veneers

1. Question: How many visits do porcelain veneers take to do?

Answer: *Porcelain veneers are placed in two visits. Whether you have one veneer or twenty eight, it is still a two-visit procedure*

2. Question: What will I look like between visits – can I go to work?

Answer: *If your veneers are being placed by an experienced cosmetic dentist, temporary bonded veneers will be placed after the first visit. They will look more than adequate for you to go about your daily routine. They will not be flossable since they will be fused together for added retention. You should not judge your final product by the look of your temporaries.*

3. Question: Do porcelain veneers change color over time?

Answer: *Porcelain is a color stable material, just like glass. However, the cement used to fuse porcelain veneers to teeth, as well as the original underlying tooth itself, could get slightly darker with time. This may slightly influence the color of the overlying veneer. If veneers are properly maintained you should not notice any significant color shift over time.*

4. Question: Is there any special care necessary to maintain porcelain veneers?

Answer: *You must brush and floss your veneers daily. You should also have your veneers professionally cleaned by a dentist or a dental hygienist every three to four months.*

5. Question: Do porcelain veneers break easily? Will I have to watch what kind of foods I eat?

Answer: *Once porcelain veneers are fused to your natural teeth, they are extremely strong. However, there are foods that can break porcelain veneers, just as they would your own natural teeth. These include: chewing on bones, biting extremely hard candies, chewing extremely hard nuts, crunching ice cubes, and chewing very hard pretzels. If you use common sense when choosing foods, your veneers will not break and will provide years of service.*

6. Question: How long will porcelain veneers last?

Answer: *Typically, porcelain veneers should last a minimum of ten years or more, if placed by an experienced cosmetic dentist. In my practice, over 95% of all veneers placed fifteen years ago are still functioning and look beautiful today.*

7. Question: Are there any guarantees with porcelain veneers?

Answer: *Most state laws prohibit any health care professionals from guaranteeing any biologic procedure. This law exists because local and systemic biology can change rapidly, affecting any previously performed biologic procedure. Simply stated, a healthy tooth, as well as a properly restored tooth, could develop future problems.*

Since porcelain veneers are expensive, most cosmetic dentists will replace any veneer that breaks within three years of its original placement, providing that the patient is maintaining the veneers (through regular hygiene) in the office where the veneers were placed.

8. Question: Can veneers be placed over existing crowns and bridges?

Answer: *If the crowns or bridges are made from porcelain, the answer is yes, provided that the crowns or bridges still fit the underlying tooth structure well.*

9. Question: Do porcelain veneers cause gum problems?

Answer: *Because porcelain veneers are extremely thin and do not go into the gum tissue, gum problems rarely develop.*

Traditionally, all porcelain margins are tolerated by the periodontal tissues much better than other dental materials.

10. Question: Can porcelain veneers be placed on teeth that have had root canal?

Answer: *Yes, provided that a ceramic post is placed within the tooth first and adequate tooth structure remains to support the veneer.*

11. Question: How old do you have to be to have porcelain veneers?

Answer: *You must be old enough so that your bony facial anatomy has stopped growing. This typically occurs between ages 16 and 18.*

12. Question: Can I just place veneers on my upper teeth and not the lowers? How will that look?

Answer: *Many people have porcelain veneers placed just on their upper teeth, and then just bleach their lower teeth. A slight color discrepancy between arches will appear. If a proper veneer color is chosen, the bleached teeth will blend enough to create a pleasing smile.*

13. Question: Can veneers be placed without preparing (drilling) the original tooth underneath?

Answer: *In rare instances, veneers can be placed on teeth without any drilling or tooth preparation. In most situations, however, the teeth would appear too bulky from the layered materials if the underlying teeth are not reduced. It is better to reduce a minimal amount of tooth structure and replace that exact amount with porcelain, so that in the final product the teeth look as natural as possible.*

14. Question: I hear and read of so many different kinds of veneers in magazines and on TV. Which veneers are the best?

Answer: *The names of veneers are just that – 'brand' names. Different dental laboratories call their veneers by different names in an attempt to influence the public perception so as to increase their market share. Be careful of all the hype. There are many, many dental laboratories that fabricate excellent porcelain veneers. The bottom line is individual talent and experience. If you have a very experienced and talented cosmetic dentist, who is using a very experienced and talented ceramist, your final veneers will turn out natural and beautiful. Don't shop 'brand names' – shop for talent and experience.*

15. Question: What if I don't like my veneers when they arrive? Can they be changed?

Answer: Absolutely, yes. The key is to try in the veneers and carefully examine them before they are permanently fused to your teeth. If changes and corrections are to be made, this is the time to request them. Once they are permanently fused to your teeth, they cannot be changed.

16. Question: What will my teeth feel like after the veneers are placed? Will I have difficulty getting used to them?

Answer: Your teeth should feel natural and normal after your veneers are placed. The highly glazed surface mimics natural tooth structure. If your bite does not feel right, have your dentist adjust it until it feels absolutely correct. Your mouth should feel exactly as it did before veneer placement.

17 Question: Can veneers be removed and would I be able to go back to my original teeth?

Answer: No. Once veneers are placed, this is a permanent cosmetic dental procedure. Veneers can only be replaced by other veneers or by crowns.

18. Question: Will my teeth be sensitive after my veneers are placed?

Answer: Your teeth should feel absolutely normal after placement. In very rare instances, some teeth may be slightly sensitive to cold temperatures. This should dissipate within two weeks.

19. Question: Will veneers make my teeth look strange under a black light at a nightclub or bar?

Answer: Veneers made with quality porcelain do not look strange under black light.

20. Question: Will my veneers look different in pictures?

Answer: Veneers tend to appear whiter in photographs than they actually appear in person. This is due to the reflective properties of flash photography.

Common Teeth Whitening and Bleaching Questions

1. Question: What are the different ways to bleach my teeth?

Answer: The first way to bleach your teeth is a 'one visit' procedure that takes about an hour in a dentist's office. The second way is to have custom trays made by a dentist for home bleaching. The third way is by purchasing 'over the counter' bleaching strips. In my opinion, the best way is the one hour office procedure, followed by custom tray bleaching at home to increase and maintain shade brightness over time.

2. Question: Does bleaching hurt?

Answer: Some people experience sensitivity during and after the bleaching procedure. In rare instances, this can last up to several weeks. If sensitivity occurs, it is usually gone within forty-eight hours.

3. Question: Does bleaching soften or damage my teeth?

Answer: All dental research confirms that using ADA approved bleaching agents do not soften or damage teeth in any way.

4. Question: Will bleached teeth fade over time?

Answer: All bleached teeth will fade with time. Color fading occurs within three to six months after bleaching. For this reason, most

cosmetic dentists provide the patients with a custom touch up tray to maintain color, or bring color back if it shifts.

5. Question: How white can your teeth be bleached?

Answer: First of all, teeth get 'brighter', more than they get 'whiter'. People with different color teeth respond differently to bleaching. Yellow teeth respond the best, while brown or gray teeth tend to respond poorly. Intrinsically stained teeth, such as tetracycline stains, will not bleach well at all.

6. Question: Is there anything else I should know before I bleach my teeth?

Answer: Prior to bleaching, you should have a recent set of x-rays and an oral exam by a dentist. This is to assure that there is no decay or gum disease present, which would need to be addressed before you bleach.

7. Question: Are there any medical considerations before bleaching teeth?

Answer: Yes, certain medications cannot be taken before or during bleaching. Temporary tooth and gum sensitivity may occur. Read manufacturer informed consent clearly. Discuss potential problems with your cosmetic dentist.

8. Question: Will tooth colored fillings or porcelain crowns be affected by the tooth bleaching process?

Answer: *No, they will remain the same color. However, if many differently colored dental materials are in the mouth prior to bleaching, they may appear dramatically different or not match the teeth that are bleached. You actually may have to change the tooth colored fillings after bleaching for a pleasing cosmetic result.*

9. Question: Do I have to avoid any types of food or drinks after bleaching?

Answer: *Yes, you must consume only bland colored foods for at least forty-eight hours. No coffee, tea, tomato sauce, berries, carrot juice, red wine, or any foods or beverages that typically stain teeth. A good rule of thumb is to eat only 'white' food- mashed potatoes, rice, bread, milk, etc. for at least two days. Use common sense in your long term diet.*

10. Question: Is there a special toothpaste required after bleaching?

Answer: *A toothpaste containing a tooth whitener or bleaching agent would be your best choice if you want to maintain the brightest look possible. These are available over the counter.*

Common Questions asked About Dental Implants

1. Question: Is the dental implant procedure painful?

Answer: *No. Local anesthesia is more than adequate to numb and eliminate the pain during the procedure. There should be absolutely no pain associated with dental implant placement.*

2. Question: Who can place a dental implant?

Answer: *Any dentist trained in advanced dental implant surgery can place an implant. Implant dentists are listed in the American Academy of Implant Dentistry directory. Typically, a 'fellow' in the academy will have*

151

more experience in implant placement. Board certified periodontists and oral surgeons, who are not members of this academy, may also be qualified to place dental implants.

3. Question: Are there any age limitations for placing dental implants?

Answer: *Anyone above the age of 18 years old who is in generally good health is a potential candidate for dental implants.*

4. Question: How long do implants last?

Answer*: If the dental implant 'takes', or osseointegrates into the bone, implants can last 20+ years. Many times dental implants will last the entire lifetime of the patient.*

5. Question: Are there any special maintenance requirements for dental implants?

Answer: *Yes, you must brush and floss your teeth daily, and have your teeth professionally cleaned by a dentist or dental hygienist three to four times per year.*

6. Question: Can dental implants be 'rejected'?

Answer: *Yes. If dental implants are rejected, this usually occurs within two to three months of placement. If implants are stable after one year, they typically last a very, very long time.*

7. Question: What causes dental implants to fail?

Answer: *The most common cause of dental implant failure is smoking cigarettes. Cigarette smoking will decrease implant prognosis by as much as 50%. Uncontrolled diabetes is another cause of dental implant failure. Other factors contributing to dental implant failures are poor oral hygiene, poor diet, systemic illnesses, and poorly constructed restorations above the implant.*

8. Question: How long does the dental implant restoration process take?

Answer: *After dental implants are placed, they should be allowed to heal for at least four months. After this initial healing period, the dental implants can be restored with either fixed teeth, or with removable overdenture type teeth. Depending upon the complexity of the restoration, it can take several additional months to complete.*

9. Question: Does dental insurance cover dental implants?

Answer: *There are a few exceptions, but usually insurance companies do not cover dental implants. Ask your benefits provider for the specifics of your dental insurance policy.*

10. Question: Can anyone get dental implants?

Answer: *No. Besides health concerns, there are local factors in the mouth which may preclude someone from getting dental implants. These include the quality and quantity of the available bone for implant placement. Other factors such as nerves, blood vessels, cysts or sinus' may also influence implant placement.*

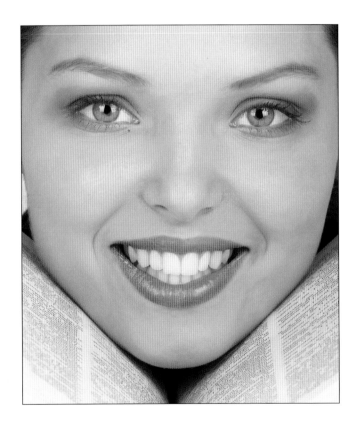

NOW IT'S YOUR TURN

There has been a dramatic rise in cosmetic dentistry procedures throughout the United States in recent years. This dramatic interest is the result of public realization that a beautiful smile is attractive, thanks in large part to Hollywood makeover shows and Madison Avenue. But an attractive smile projects more than beauty, according to studies conducted by the American Academy of Cosmetic Dentistry. It also projects to others a sense of intelligence, confidence, interesting personality, success, friendliness, happiness and wealth as well.

Anyone can have a great looking smile. The first step to achieving the ideal smile is recognizing that shame and embarrassment over the appearance of one's teeth can be easily overcome. Many patients claim that they forgot how to smile naturally. Some avoid being photographed because of their teeth and cover their mouth with their hands when they smile, dodge kissing and even steer clear of situations that require speaking in front of others. The number of people suffering from a lack of self-esteem because of their smile has reached epidemic proportions. This may account for the sudden surge in the interest in cosmetic dentistry. Self-consciousness and/or discontent with one's smile leads to a lack of confidence which leads to unhappiness which leads to an overall negative body image. The good news is—you can change all of this.

Most of the procedures necessary to correct the problems of aesthetically imperfect teeth are not difficult, painful or time-consuming to perform. The three barriers to making a commitment to have the procedures done are lack of information, procrastination, and fear. "I thought nothing could be done, otherwise someone would have suggested I do something about it" and "Someday I'm going to have my teeth fixed" are typical responses. Others believe it will be a painful procedure or they may fear they can't afford it. Others fear that the results may not meet their expectations.

Lack of information should no longer be an excuse. This book contains all the information you need to know to seek answers on how to address your specific concerns. Don't be surprised by not receiving advice from those around you. It is difficult for family and friends to feel comfortable telling someone they care about that their smile needs improvement. The bottom line is, you know that your smile needs improvement. Why not correct it? It is not difficult to do. In fact, there are easy solutions for smile enhancement that may be life changing events.

Procrastination does nothing but prolong the unnecessary agony of not being able to smile comfortably. The first step is recognizing the problem. The next step is finding out what can be done about it. It is important to find a cosmetic dentist you can trust and who makes you feel comfortable. Together you will work out a game plan to create a beautiful smile that will change your life.

Patients no longer need to be fearful. State-of-the-art cosmetic dental procedures are painless. There are numerous financial options available that make a new smile affordable for almost anyone. As far as results, cosmetic dental procedures are very predictable if good communication exists between the cosmetic dentist and patient. This is made even easier with advances in computer simulation and chairside mock-up techniques.

Communication is essential. Excellent, sound dental treatment is enhanced when clear, concise communication exists between patient and dentist.

Cosmetic dentistry can be expensive, but finances should never be a barrier. There are many creative solutions available for having cosmetic dental procedures performed – procedures that are deserved by anyone who needs them.

Age is not a barrier. There is no such thing as being too old to look beautiful.

A great smile increases confidence and will enhance your communication skills. For the career minded person, this creates a competitive edge in job performance. The truth is that everyone can use this competitive psychological edge, whether in the work place or socially. When asked what features are most alluring in a person, most people will put a great looking smile on the top of their list. Shouldn't it be at the top of yours when you think about yourself?

Find out how powerful and magnetic a great looking smile will be for you. Your smile can change your life. You must have the courage to make the decision NOW to improve the way you look.

This can be a whole new beginning for you. I challenge you not to make any more excuses or procrastinate any longer. You can do it! Find a cosmetic dentist. Discover the thrill and excitement that a new smile through cosmetic dentistry can bring to your life.

You deserve an Amazing Smile!

155

To order more copies of this book visit
AmazingSmilesBook.com

ALBERT J. KURPIS, D.D.S.

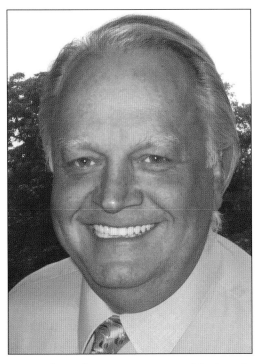

Dr. Albert J. Kurpis received his dental degree from Columbia University, College of Dental Medicine in 1974. He was immediately invited back to teach future dentists the art and science of advanced restorative and prosthetic dentistry. He maintained his associate professorship there until the mid nineteen eighties. It was from here that his life long work in the field of cosmetic dentistry and dental implantology began. His early research with baboon primates culminated in a dental implant design so unique that the United States government granted him a patent for his work.

Dr. Kurpis has taught dental implant techniques and cosmetic dental procedures to thousands of dentists in the United States, Europe, and the Middle East. He has served in many prestigious professional organizations as well as being past president of the northeast section of the American Academy of Implant Dentistry. He is a member of the American Academy of Cosmetic Dentistry, Greater New York Academy of Prosthodontics and a member of numerous other prestigious dental organizations. He has been seen on many television programs, national magazines, and radio talk shows. He has published numerous articles in both professional and consumer journals and continues to help other dentists, consulting in the field of cosmetic and implant dentistry. He holds a dental license in New York, New Jersey and California. Yet, with a prolific background, he still enjoys serving his patients as a clinician in his beautiful state-of-the-art cosmetic dental office located in Ridgewood, New Jersey.

For more information, Dr. Kurpis can be reached at (201) 447-9700.

Additional information on his work and cosmetic dentistry procedures
can be found at his website located at:

CosmeticDentist.com